STRESS AND GENERAL PRACTITIONERS

by

Usha Rout
Lecturer in Psychology, Manchester Metropolitan University, Manchester, UK

and

Jaya K. Rout
General Practitioner, Bolton, UK

KLUWER ACADEMIC PUBLISHERS
DORDRECHT / BOSTON / LONDON

Distributors

for the United States and Canada: Kluwer Academic Publishers, PO Box 358, Accord Station, Hingham, MA 02018-0358, USA
for all other countries: Kluwer Academic Publishers Group, Distribution Center, PO Box 322, 3300 AH Dordrecht, The Netherlands

ISBN 0-7923-8815-1

A catalogue record for this book is available from the British Library.

Published in the United Kingdom by Kluwer Academic Publishers, PO Box 55, Lancaster, UK.

Kluwer Academic Publishers BV incorporates the publishing programmes of D. Reidel, Martinus Nijhoff, Dr W. Junk and MTP Press.

Printed and bound in Great Britain by Cromwell Press, Melksham, Wilts.

Contents

Preface

General practice has taken on a new shape since the introduction of the new contract for GPs in April 1990, one of the most radical changes in the profession for many years. The initial widespread dissent from many GPs, widely publicised in the media, has now more or less disappeared. But there is no doubt that GPs work patterns have changed quite radically and will continue to do so. This is especially so in the area of management – a field that many still find it difficult to get to grips with and this area is likely to be a growing problem as further changes, such as fund holding occur. Yet there has been no quantitative research on how GPs have coped with these radical changes in their working life and in particular their effect on stress in the profession.

Stress is present in all professions; stress related diseases such as heart disease, anxiety, depression, and alcohol and drug abuse are well documented. Yet there is surprisingly little written about the profession that often has to deal with the end-results of stress – GPs.

The work described in this book was inspired by the lack of any British studies on stress and stress outcomes in doctors in general and GPs in particular. The few studies in Britain have focused on junior doctors and medical students; there has been no large scale study on stress in GPs.

Chapter 1 describes briefly the background to the NHS and the recent changes that have affected the work of the GP. Chapters 2, 3 and 4 give an overview of what stress is and a review of the available literature on stress in the medical profession.

Chapters 5, 6 and 7 describe our two studies on stress and GPs. The first of these chapters highlights some of the qualitative material extracted from interviews with GPs before the introduction of the new contract. The main study, a postal survey of over 1800 GPs also carried our before the introduction of the new contract, is described in the other two chapters. Finally in Chapter 8 we briefly mention our post-contract qualitative study and then we review some of the important issues of stress management and coping strategies that GPs may find valuable.

Although there have been many books on stress in other professions there is no general book on stress and methods of coping with it in general practice that can be used by GPs, trainee GPs and medical students. Also this book may be used by researchers interested in this area. We hope that this book goes some way to rectifying this situation and provides the reader with an overview of stress among GPs as well as a stimulus for further research in this important field.

Although we have, as far as possible, attempted to present a fair and unbiased view of the subject it is inevitable that in a book of this nature the views of the authors will come through. We are a husband and wife team, a GP and a psychologist, whose life very much revolves around general practice and the study of stress in it! We are happy to accept that there will be criticisms from those whose views strongly contradict ours but hope that this book will stimulate further debate on what we believe is an area of growing importance in medicine in general and general practice in particular.

Throughout the book we have, for the sake of simplicity, followed the convention of using the masculine article unless specifically discussing gender. We are not unaware that a significant and growing proportion of doctors is female and hope that this usage will not give offence.

Acknowledgements

Our nationwide study was only possible due to the cooperation of all those GPs who were willing to give up their valuable time in completing lengthy questionnaires and taking part in interviews. Our fear that British GPs would be secretive in expressing their feelings was proved wrong and we hope that this book verifies the inner feelings of many. We would like to thank Professor Cary Cooper, for his guidance and support during the precontract research. We would also like to thank our colleagues, Professor Paul Iles and Dr Carolyn Kagan who have provided useful comments and criticism that we have, wherever possible, tried to incorporate. Finally we would like to thank our son Tony and daughter Natalie for their patience. The final content of the book is however, our sole responsibility.

Commonly used abbreviations

BMA: British Medical Association
DH: Department of Health
DHSS: Department of Health and Social Security
DSS: Department of Social Security
FHSA: Family Health Services Authority
FPC: Family Practitioner Committee
GMC: General Medical Council
GMSC: General Medical Services Committee
GP(s): General Practitioner(s)
NHS: National Health Service
PGEA: Post Graduate Education Allowance
RCGP: Royal College of General Practitioners
LMC: Local Medical Committee
NASS: National Association for Staff Support
AAFP: American Academy of Family Physicians

Chapter 1 – INTRODUCTION AND BACKGROUND

This chapter describes briefly the background to the National Health Service (NHS) and the recent changes that have affected the working patterns of GPs. It will also help those readers unfamiliar with the organisation of the NHS and the profession of General Practice to understand these two key elements.

The development of General Practice in the NHS

The National Health Service was introduced in the United Kingdom in 1948 to provide medical care for the whole population. Primary medical care in the UK is usually provided through general practice and the vast majority of the population is registered with general practitioners (GPs). The GP is in the front line of the NHS and is the first point of contact with the health service for most people seeking medical advice. In the UK provision of patient care by means of general practice is provided in the centre of cities, in towns, in the country and even on remote islands.

The role of the GP in the UK may be different from the equivalent doctor in other countries in that they provide medical care in surgeries, at the patient's home and sometimes also in hospitals. Patients have direct access to their GP without any other referral. This enhances contact with the patient population. GPs may then refer their patients to any other part of the NHS as they deem to be advisable. No other profession can claim to have contact with two-thirds of the population over a one-year period [1].

The definition agreed by the Leeuwenhorst group [2] of the GPs job and accepted by most people today is:

> "The GP is a licenced medical graduate who gives personal, primary and continuing care to individuals, families and a practice population irrespective of age, sex and illness. It is the synthesis of these functions which is unique. He will attend his patients in his consulting room and in their homes and sometimes in a clinic or hospital. His aim is to make early diagnosis. He will include and integrate physical, psychological and social factors in his considerations about health and illness . . . He will make an initial decision about every problem presented to him as a doctor. He will undertake to continuing management of patients with chronic, recurrent or terminal illnesses . . . He will practice in cooperation with other colleagues, medical and non-medical."

It is important to note that GPs are not employed directly by the health service, but are classified as self-employed individuals contracted to the NHS. Their contracts require them to provide care for all people who are registered with them. They earn their income essentially from 'basic practice allowances', capitation fees payable for each patient and items of service (i.e. immunisation, delivery, post-natal care, provision of contraception, IUD, etc.). There are other supplementary allowances paid to GP practices for such things as construction and improvement of premises and reimbursement of salary costs of ancillary and nursing staff.

During the 1950s and early 1960s general practice remained an unattractive career option for junior doctors. Most of the technological facilities of the hospitals were unavailable to GPs, and the status of GPs was low. An ambitious medical graduate seemingly had only one suitable choice to follow – a career in hospital medicine. There were attempts to shift the balance. The Cohen Committee [3] called for a three-year vocational training scheme for GPs. Entry into general practice from the early 1970s was usually by vocational training. This became mandatory in 1982. The College of General Practitioners (later to become the Royal College (RCGP)), was established in 1952 and the first academic Department of General Practice was founded in 1957 in Edinburgh.

During the 1960s general practice was an unpopular career choice according to a survey conducted by Last and Stanley [4]. Although certain studies [5,6] have shown an increase in the popularity of general practice among medical students, variations between medical schools seems to suggest that different teachers may have influenced career choices. Over the past two decades the status of general practice changed. It moved from being one of the least to one of the most popular career choices for newly qualified doctors in comparison with the low pay and competitive tensions of a hospital career. This trend appears to be changing, however, following the introduction of the new contract for GPs [7].

Whilst the pattern of medical education in general seems to be continued to be dominated by doctor controlled, disease centered 'expert medicine' this is being challenged by general practice teaching which emphasises the importance of dealing with the social and psychological rather than the physical aspects of medicine. Communication skills and the management of uncertainty in general practice is now beginning to be taught during medical training.

General practice has gradually changed over the past twenty years from solo practices to group practices (Tables 1.1 and 1.2). After pressure from the British Medical Association, direct financial incentives for group practice were provided in the family doctor's 'charter' in 1966. The British Medical Association Board of Science and Education [8] has stressed the advantages of group practice. They pointed out that peer influence and informal learning within the group raise the status of the GP; hence GPs may find their work more satisfying. Doctors in a group practice can afford to have better premises and equipment and more ancillary staff than a single-handed GP.

Cartwright and Anderson [9] in their study found that doctors practising in group tend to be of younger age group than those of single-handed doctors. As more young doctors enter into group practices this influx in future may enhance its status. Also it was found by the same authors that GPs practising from groups have a more even distribution of work, have better equipped practice premises, more ancillary staff, and have the time to take outside part-time work.

Table 1.1 Changes in the size of partnerships

	Percentage of GPs				
Type of practice	1951	1961	1971	1977	1981
Single-handed practices	43	28	20	16	13
Two partners	38	34	24	20	18
Three partners	13	21	25	24	22
Four partners	5	11	17	19	19
Five partners	1	4	8	12	14
Six or more partners	–	2	6	9	14
Total (%)	100	100	100	100	100
Total number of unrestricted principals		18905	19374	20796	

Source: Department of Health and Social Security. Health and Personal Social Services Statistics for England, 1978, London: HMSO, 1980, Health and Personal Social Services Statistics, 1982, Table 3.22

The trend towards larger practices has continued, so that the proportion of doctors in practices with three or more partners has increased from 42% in 1964 to 60% in 1973 [11]. Tables 1.1 and 1.2 show the growth of partnership from 1951–1981 and 1969–1990. Also in the five years from 1968 to 1973 the number of whole time equivalent clerical staff went up by 10% each year and the number of employed nurses by 26% overall [12]. A new concept of primary health care team began to emerge [13]. GPs were no longer expected to work in isolation, but in collaboration with other health professionals to provide overall health care in the community.

The primary health care team of the 1990s is usually composed of GPs, practice managers, secretarial staff, practice nurses, and staff employed by the area health authority such as health visitors, midwives, and district nurses. Social workers are also occasionally attached by the local authority. Less frequently, other staff, such as physiotherapists, psychologists, or chiropodists, may attend a surgery for certain sessions. As practices get bigger organisational problems increase, and the requirement for communication and consultation between the members of the practice (e.g. partners, employees and attached staff) increases too.

Table 1.2. General medical practitioners: analysis by type of practice

	1969	1979	1984	1985	1986	1987	1988	1989	1990
All practitioners: Total	20208	23062	25788	26190	26529	27023	27420	27749	27523
Unrestricted principals:									
Total	18901	21357	23640	24035	24460	24922	25322	25608	25622
Single-handed	4131	3179	2926	2915	2926	2875	2915	2929	2975
In partnership of:									
2 doctors	4828	4054	3866	3880	3824	3860	3885	3827	3865
3 doctors	4875	5096	5103	4986	4976	4902	4750	4702	4581
4 doctors	2876	4112	4288	4352	4390	4448	4588	4655	4543
5 doctors	1290	2600	3490	3610	3805	3835	3889	3960	4107
6 or more doctors	898	2316	3967	4292	4539	5002	5295	5535	5551

Source: [10]

The number of GPs in the NHS is increasing (Table 1.2). In a district of 250,000 persons there is an average of 120 GPs. The practices are in varying sizes, approximately one GP to 2100 persons. In a practice with 2500 persons registered with the NHS the likely work profile can be expressed by division of the various activities [14]:

- consultation and home visits 65%
- patient services (letters, phone, prescriptions) 15%
- practice administration 8%
- other professional activities 12%

The question may be raised as to whether there is an ideal list size. Little research has been carried out on how many patients a doctor can reasonably be expected to provide comprehensive care. It involves examination of resources, quality of care as well as practice organisation and staffing levels.

Recent changes in the NHS – 'the new GP contract' and the implications of the changes

The White Paper 'Promoting Better Health', published in 1988, proposed several changes in GPs' terms of service and remuneration. Agreement was reached on the major issues of the White Paper following consultation with representatives of the profession. Subsequently the profession rejected the representatives' support for the change but the Government believes that it was the best way forward for improving services to patients and for rewarding those GPs who provided the best service. The 'New Contract' was introduced on 1 April 1990. The key points in the Government's plan to improve general medical service were:

1. giving patients better choice by providing them with more information about the services GPs offer. There will be more competition, and it will be made easier to change doctors

2. making the terms of service more specific to reflect clearly the requirements of good general practice that better practices already meet in serving their patients

3. amending the Statement of Fees and Allowances (SFA) so that the remuneration system becomes more performance related, enabling GPs who provide high quality services to be better paid

4. strengthening the contractual relationship with Family Practitioner Committees and Health Boards in Scotland to encourage the provision of good quality services

5. ensuring that there is greater value for money in the general medical services [15].

In an organisation change can be expected to occur all the time and can be regarded as a necessity. But if such change is brought about at an accelerated rate without taking into consideration the human capacity to cope with it, it may produce shock and the inability to adjust. When change occurs as a perceived need it is more likely to be appreciated and less likely to be rejected. If change is imposed from outside without prior agreed consultation and without supporting pilot studies then the members of the organisation may feel victimised. Changes imposed by others may be considered to be tyrannical and can cause a sense of hopelessness and helplessness.

The new GP contract appears to be a clear example of imposed changes: there is no empirical research or evidence in support of the change. These changes constituted the most significant alteration in the structure, standards and attitude of general practice since the implementation of the 1965 charter. The main areas of change involved target settings for immunisation, cervical cytology, health promotion clinics, minor surgery, invitations to patients not seen within the last three years, screening of elderly patients, night visits, seniority payments, post-graduate education allowances (PGEA) and prescribing.

Administrative changes included criteria for ancillary staff employment, practice leaflets, annual reports, audit, fund holding and buying local hospital services. We shall look briefly at some of these items in more detail.

Cervical cytology

According to the new contractual arrangements GPs are no longer paid individually for cervical cytology tests, but payment is based on a system of target payments based on specified levels of uptake. A GP receives a target payment at the higher rate if he achieves an uptake of 80% and at a lower rate if at least 50% of eligible women have had adequate smears. The target calculation does not take into account the women who either do not wish to have cervical smears or those who refuse. Hence some GPs may find it difficult to achieve their targets.

Immunization for children aged 2 and under

The new contract provides for a target payment system to replace the previous arrangement of individual payment for each immunization provided to children under the age of 2.

A GP is eligible for a target payment at the higher rate if, on the first day of the quarter, the number of courses completed amount to 90% and for a target payment at the lower rate if the average of courses completed amounts to 70% of the numbers needed for full immunization. But the problem is that this does not take into account those who cannot be immunized due to some medical reasons or whose parents do not wish their children to be immunized.

Seniority and PGEA

Seniority payments to GPs who have completed the prescribed years of registration with the General Medical Council (GMC) and worked as unrestricted NHS GPs are retained but the amount paid is reduced to be compensated for by the new PGEA. To be eligible for PGEA a GP has to provide evidence that they have attended an average of 30 hours accredited post-graduate education a year over the past five years. Many GPs may now have to travel long distances to meet their PGEA requirements at the cost of their family and social life. As one GP's wife said:

> ". . . A new game has evolved – chasing PGEA sessions. That means a boring evening out for a half-session, and a waste of a lunch time for a third. I thought that once senior partner status was reached things would be different. But now I find meeting after meeting eroding our time together. I did not perceive life as a doctor's wife being like this" [16].

The question has been raised whether there is a genuine interest to learn any academic facts from such meetings or just to sign the register to obtain accreditation to fulfill PGEA requirements.

Night visits

There are two levels of payments for visits carried out between 10 pm and 8 am: a lower fee is paid if a visit is made by a deputizing doctor and a higher fee if visited by the patient's own GP, his partner or a member of an approved group. The attraction of a higher fee and avoidance of payment to the deputising service may tempt a GP to conduct the night visits himself but lack of sleep may cause impairment in clinical judgement.

As one GP has been quoted as saying:

> "Why has the Government insisted on these changes? The most charitable argument might be that it necessarily believes it is better for patients if their GP does his or her own night work. But care which might benefit someone at 3 a.m. will certainly be to the detriment of 20, 30 or more people the next day [17]."

Prescribing

The FHSAs through their medical advisors are involved in GP prescribing. They cooperate with District Health Authorities to establish rational prescribing and develop mechanisms to monitor individual doctors prescribing habits and investigate excessive prescribing. Indicative prescribing, a system whereby a GP 'indicates' the expected spending on prescribed drugs, is also being introduced.

We believe that unless a uniform policy and attitude is applied to all sections of the NHS it may not be easy for GPs to stay within their allocated budgets. It would seem that in some cases hospitals are requesting GPs to prescribe expensive drugs to patients because the hospital would not be allowed to prescribe such drugs from their own budget. One GP described his dilemma and problem with regard to prescribing:

> "The information indicating our prescribing budget for this coming financial year is ludicrous. We just couldn't possibly keep up with it though we are average prescribers. We're being given less than we prescribed last year [18]."

Fund holding

The government's intentions of reform of the NHS is to make it 'more business like' and therefore provide a better health care to the nation although it has been voiced by many GPs that doctors are clinicians and not accountants. One aspect of this has been to allow certain group practices to operate as small businesses 'buying' services from health care providers using an annual budget – fund holding.

The objectives of fund holding are:

- To improve the quality of services on offer to patients by GPs
- To help GPs develop their practices for the benefit of their patients.
- To allow GPs greater control over the use of resources for their patients
- To encourage hospitals to be more responsive to the need of GPs and their patients [19].

Those doctors who have opted for fund holding may be good at accounting or may have taken the option for a trial period, but a large majority of GPs remain opposed to the idea of fund holding. Some fund holding GPs have now resigned from their jobs after noticing development of mistrust by their patients. As one GP said:

> "I think fund holding is a misleading feature of the new GP contract. I can no longer afford to practice medicine where my patients confidence and trust of me is eroded now. I am resigning."

Patients also have started asking 'are you prescribing these cheaper drugs because you are a fund holder?' It has also been claimed that fund holding will create a two-tier health service with patients of fund holders receiving better or faster treatment than the rest of the population.

Fund holding involves numerous meetings with practice members, regional health authority coordinators, FHSA members and health care providers units which are extremely time-consuming and some of them may be unproductive. Too many meetings are adding to the GPs' time pressure and worsening their stress levels.

The intensity of a GP's work load has also increased. To quote a GP:

> "The analogy I use is that you can spend an hour sprinting flat out or strolling gently. Both of them could be described as moving from A to B. My experience of general practice is that, pretty well everyday now, it's sprinting flat out. The day is just not long enough to do what we've got to do." [20]

Chapter 2 – WHAT IS STRESS?

In this chapter we briefly describe the concept and definition of stress and highlight alternative approaches to the study of stress. Also 'burn out' and coping strategies are concisely portrayed.

Understanding stress

Nowadays, stress has increasingly become a part of our everyday vocabulary. We hear about it on radio, on television, in newspapers, and at conferences. Yet, there is division of opinion about the proper use of the term stress. The word stress (derived from Latin) was used popularly in the seventeeth century to mean hardship, straits, adversity or affliction [21]. During the eighteenth century its use evolved to denote 'force, pressure, strain or strong effort', with reference mainly to a person or person's organs or mental powers. In 1910, William Osler suggested that there was a causal relationship between hardwork, stress and strain with his patients suffering from 'Angina Pectoris'. Walter Cannon [22] proposed the 'fight or flight response' of an organism to its environment; when the stressor (environmental event that results in stress) comes from outside, one may attempt to fight (resist) at these times, while at other times one may attempt to escape (run away) from it. He emphasised the stimulation of sympathetic nervous system, with the resulting hormonal discharge from the adrenal glands, which occurs during emergencies such as pain. This autonomic process induces the cardiovascular changes that prepare the body for flight or fight.

Stress has been used to refer to environmental circumstances that disrupt the normal activity of an organism [23]. It has also referred to the responses of the organism, either physiological or psychological to particular events [24–26] or as an overall label for a field of study that examines the process by which organisms adapt to disruptive events [27]. Selye [28] was one of the first to introduce the concept of stress into the life sciences. Some of the relevant aspects of Selye's development of the stress concept will now be outlined.

Selye [29] defined stress as 'a non-specific defensive and adaptive mechanism arising out of exposure to a stressor'. A stressor for Selye is not necessarily a noxious experience. The demands or agents that evoke the patterned or standard response are referred to as stressors. According to this view, any demand made on the body elicits a demand for readjustment for homoeostasis. A person is never free from the demands made on him by his environment and is constantly engaged in life maintaining activity of some sort. Selye emphasized this by stating that 'complete freedom from stress is death' [30]. He states that it makes no difference whether the stress is negative (e.g. divorce, loss of a job, death of a spouse) or positive (e.g. winning an award, advancing on the job, receiving a salary increase). Positive and negative stressors produce the same physiological reaction [25].

According to Selye [30] the non-specific response of the body to any demand is manifested through the General Adaptation Syndrome (GAS) which develops in three stages:

1. Alarm reaction: when an organism is exposed to an unadapted stimulus there is an initial shock (in which resistance is lowered) followed by a rebound reaction (counter shock phase) during which the organism's defence mechanisms become active.

2. Stage of resistance: during this stage the organism's full adaptation may lead to successful return to equilibrium. However, if the stressor continues or the defence does not work, he will move onto the final stage.

3. Stage of exhaustion: in case of failure of adaptability the organism becomes exhausted which leads to terminality.

He claims that the above three stages are not as distinct as they may look on paper. They are artificial divisions of what in real life is a continuous process. The transition from one to another is gradual. According to Selye's view although the aim of the GAS is to maintain homoeostasis, prolonged adaptive effort can be counter-productive and give rise to 'diseases of adaptation', i.e. stress diseases. These diseases will differ between individuals because each person is genetically disposed to be weaker in one bodily organ or system than in others; or psycho-social factors may differ. One person, for example, may respond to stress by increasing his or her intake of alcohol whereas another may adapt by becoming increasingly obsessional. Selye's view is that:

> "The justification for calling any malady a disease of adaptation is directly proportional to the role that maladjustment to stress plays in its development . . . typical diseases of adaptation are due to insufficient, excessive or faulty reactions to stressors, as an inappropriate hormonal or nervous responses. Thus, the term should be used only when the maladaptation factor appears to be more important than the eliciting pathogen itself." [30]

It is not necessary for all three stages of GAS to develop; only the most severe stress leads rapidly to the stage of exhaustion. Most of the stressors that act upon an individual during a limited period produce changes corresponding only to the first and second stages. At first the stressors may upset and alarm the individual, but then he adapts to them.

Selye [25] views stress as essential to the life process and that alarm reactions are unavoidable. He distinguishes between good stress (positive stress) and bad stress or distress – an unpleasant feeling (harmful). The former is sometimes called eustress (from the Greek word eu meaning good) [30] and signals for coping are required. But the latter is harmful where the individual is unable to cope and enters the final phase (exhaustion) of the GAS.

Selye's theory, derived from the biological sciences, has provided the basis for more specific definitions based on psychological responses. These have used the concept of homoeostasis which is implied in the 'imbalance' that arises when demands on the individual exceed his capacity to respond. For example, Mechanic [31] defines stress as: "a discrepancy between a problem or challenge and the individuals capacity to deal or to accommodate to it".

Cox [32], reviewed the literature on alternative theoretical approaches to the study of stress and identified three major approaches.

1. *Stress as a response (a dependent variable)*

Stress is described as the response to disturbing stimuli (situation or environment). This approach is derived from Selye's writing [29,33]; stress is a state manifested by a specific syndrome which consists of all the non-specifically induced changes within a biological system [29]. This definition explains that stress is a condition of being which is manifested by a set of mechanisms (a specific syndrome) within the body. This suggests that stress results in a certain pattern of physiological changes such as gastrointestinal, glandular and cardiovascular disorders. Thus stress is non-specifically induced which means that it is caused by many different and changing agents. Moreover, it affects the entire body, not just a single part. However, Selye's concept of non-specificity has been challenged by many authors, for example, Lacey [34] and Mason [35]. Mason [35] argued that some noxious physical stimuli (for example, physical exercise, fasting, etc.) do not produce the GAS. Lacey [34] has also argued that the low intercorrelation between the various physiological indices of the GAS refute the concept of a non-specific pattern of response. Also Selye completely ignored the role of the psychological processes at work. Cox [32] suggested that much of the physiological responses are not directly determined by the actual presence of the stressors, but rather by their psychological repercussion upon the individual.

One special kind of response-based definition by McGrath [36] has received considerable attention and is based on degradation of performance. To define stress as performance degradation poses many difficulties. Many potential stressors may or may not lead to performance degradation or change in the performance. There are large differences in response within and between individuals [32]. Also all performance degradation does not arise from 'stress'; sometimes performance degradation happens for reasons of skill, motivation, etc.

2. *Stress as a stimulus (an independent variable)*

Other research has concentrated upon those stimuli that are presumed to provoke stress reactions. The more extreme proponents of this view see the sources of stress as arising solely outside the person (e.g. pressure at work or illness of a family member) and make little allowance for any intervening psychological process (e.g.

Holmes and Rahe) [37]. The life event approach [37] proposes that negative consequences of stress for health resulted more from accumulation of stressors requiring adjustment, rather than the damage by any simple one. Therefore, if too many positive or negative changes (such as marriage and divorce) occur in a very short period, they can tax the adaptive capacity of the individual and lead to increased susceptibility to mental and physical illness. This approach views stress as an independent variable for study.

This approach has been borrowed from the physical sciences, especially the field of engineering. When loads are placed on metals, they produce deformation in them due to internal strain. When the load is removed the metal will eventually return to its original condition, if the strain produced is within the 'elastic limit' of the material. If the strain crosses beyond the elastic limits, permanent damage occurs. In case of individuals stress can be tolerated up to a certain limit but thereafter permanent damage may result.

This approach has been criticised by Cox [32] as being extremely limited when it is applied to human behaviour: "men and their organisations are not machines . . . Unless the stress/strain relationship in men functions both unconsciously and automatically, we have to accept some intervening psychological process which does mediate the outcome of that relationship. Stress has to be perceived or recognised by man. A machine, however, does not have to recognise the load or stress placed upon it".

3. *Stress – an interactionist approach (stress as an intervening variable)*

Both the preceding approaches are based on a stimulus–response model (S–R). They are mechanistic, often viewing the individual as a passive recipient of stimuli from the environment. They do not take into account individual differences. For example Lazarus [38] and McGrath [36] consider that this S–R approach cannot adequately describe the stress syndrome because they do not see the importance of the individual's perception of his own reality. In adopting an interactionist approach, they emphasise the importance of the way that individuals perceive themselves and the events that impinge upon them. Therefore perception, appraisal and judgement of the situation are all important.

Lazarus [38] presents one of the well known interactionist explanations of stress. According to him "stress refers, then to a very broad class of problems differentiated from other problem areas because it deals with any demands which tax the system, whatever it is, a physiological system, a social system, or a psychological system, and the response of that system . . . depends on how the person interprets or appraises (consciously or unconsciously) the significance of a harmful, threatening or challenging event". However, Lazarus [39] has formulated a concept of cognitive appraisal and psychological stress or threat whereby stress is not seen as an imbalance between the individual's objective demand and the response capability, but an imbalance between perceived demand (or threat) and perceived response capabilities. Stress occurs not only due to external conditions but also on the person's appraisal of the situation. However, Cox [32] suggests that stress can be described as 'part of a complex and dynamic system of transaction between the person and his environment'. According to Cox, stress is "an individual perceptual phenomenon rooted in psychological processes . . . it treats stress as an intervening variable, the reflection of a transaction between the person and his environment . . ." [32].

McGrath [36] has suggested that stress occurs when there is an imbalance between environmental demand and the response capacity of the individual. According to McGrath [36], "we need to approach the problems of stress systematically with a set of concepts that encompass the full sequence of events (objective demands, subjective demands, response and consequence) and with an approach aimed at seeing the linkages among the parts of the sequence". He suggests that some of the problems of identification of 'subjective load' may be overcome by the use of multistressor, multieffect type studies.

One of the most influential of the interactionist models is the P–E (person–environment) fit model developed at the University of Michigan [40–43]. The basic idea of the P–E fit model is that 'the individual adjustment consists of the 'goodness of fit' between the characteristics of a person and the properties of the person's environment' [44]. Stress results from a mismatch (lack of fit) between an individual and his environment. In the work situation, there is emphasis on two types of fit. One is the extent to which work (the environment) provides rewards and supplies to meet individuals' needs and preferences. Misfit leads to individual strain. The other is the extent to which an individual's skills and abilities meet the demands of work. Misfit leads to organisational strain (and indirectly individual strain). Van Harrison [40] has suggested that "the basic assumption of the theory is that when misfit of either kind threatens an individual's well being, strains will occur such as job dissatisfaction, anxiety, depression and physiological problems". Hingley and Cooper [45] suggest that "the concept is particularly attractive to the researcher as it is comprehensive, it deals with the overall adjustment of the individual to their unique situation, and it has been widely used to explain the relationship between the work environment and individual well-being".

In considering occupational stress in general practice, to apply the stimulus–response model could result in dealing only with a limited proportion of the total problems of society, organisation, stress and disease. This, according to Lazarus [27], excludes other stress indices such as psychoses, neuroses, and subsequent character disorders such as alcoholism, suicide and drug addiction. It is now accepted that sources of work stress can only be adequately investigated by taking a multidisciplinary approach [46]. Hence, it must be emphasized that there is a need to investigate the whole area of problems – psychological, sociological and physiological – by which people are taxed by the stimulus demands made on them.

What is burnout?

Burnout may be defined as 'psychological withdrawal from work in response to excessive stress and dissatisfaction'. It is a state of physical, mental and emotional exhaustion. This is a special form of stress which is commonly found among those in the medical and helping professions and among administrators who have to deal a lot with people.

Three stages of burnout are recognised [47]:

1. Job stress – working excessive hours, foregoing holidays, a tendency towards hurried and skipped meals and giving little time to the family.

2. Mental or emotional exhaustion – tiredness, lethargy, hypochondria, irritability, anxiety, depression, insomnia or possibly uncontrolled alcohol consumption.

3. Inability to feel sympathy for patients. This is accompanied by a deterioration in communication skills and tardiness.

Burnout has no age limits; it can affect the young trainee or even the senior principal partner. Maslach and Jackson [48] found that burnout scores were higher for doctors who spent a greater proportion of their time with patients. Burnout doctors may work harder and harder but accomplish less and less.

People who are thought to be highly perfectionist and extremely conscientious with type A personalities (see Chapter 3) are the most vulnerable group. They have high expectations of themselves and others but are poor delegators.

Coping strategies

As yet, there is no definite statement on the meaning of coping. In simple terms, coping skills can broadly be defined as techniques for dealing with stressful demands. Coping has been defined as the process of managing external or internal demands that are perceived as taxing or exceeding a person's resources [49]. It could be recognised that coping is not only a reaction to stress; it can be preventive by anticipating a stressful situation.

The importance of coping is recently being appreciated even in those areas of psychological research where it was previously ignored. The search for good theories of coping processes, and measures of them are not as well developed as are needed to understand the consequences of stressful environments [49] but the two main functions utilised during coping are problem solving (to manage the problem causing the distress) and emotional processing (designed to regulate emotions or distress) [50].

Problem solving skills (direct action) aquired during training in medical careers may be deployed as forms of coping. Also emotional processing (palliative) such as anxiety and anxiety-reduction training may be used. Many attempts at regulating the emotions may also involve engaging in palliative coping (which focuses on regulating emotional distress and includes denial, projection, suppression, or intellectualization). Denial constitutes a refusal to accept the objective reality for what it is. It ignores the stressor. Projection is defence against our own undesirable qualities by assigning them to other people in an exaggerated manner by which means we justify ourselves in our own eyes. Suppression is the process of deliberate self control. Individuals push the painful memories (stressors) out of the way temporarily in order to concentrate on a task. Intellectualization is the process of translating feelings into thought processes. This blocks the feelings that one does not wish to deal with immediately. The problem with this process is that the individual filters out all the feelings to such an extent that he can never express his emotions. However many writers see this as the negative side of the coping process.

Table 2.1 Physical, personal and behavioural symptoms of burnout

Physical symptoms
- Fatigue
- Insomnia
- Headache
- Backache
- Gastrointestinal symptoms
- Weight gain/loss
- Shortness of breath
- Lingering cold

Personal symptoms
- Depressed
- Chronically anxious
- Obsessed
- Feeling indispensible
- Restless
- Rationalizing
- Stagnating
- Bored

Behavioural symptoms
- Irritable
- Cynical
- Defensive
- Fault finding
- Alcohol-dependent
- Drug-dependent
- Unable to enjoy others success

Source: [51]

Palliative coping leaves the origins or the source of stress unchanged, but it can make the individual feel better. There is no definite assumption here that one is better than the other. People use different methods of coping for different stressors. Problem-focused coping is especially useful for managing controllable stressors, and emotional-focused coping is suitable for managing the impact of uncontrollable stressors. In many cases people use combinations of the two in managing the demands of stressful encounters.

Coping behaviour can be described as either adaptive or maladaptive. Adaptive coping behaviour deals directly with the stressful situation by pursuing and executing solutions. Conversly, maladaptive behaviour does not deal directly with the problem faced and it is defensive in nature. Most individuals use some form of defence mechanism, (i.e. denial, projections [blaming others]), at times and in many cases it is justifiable and healthy. They help us through stressful situations until we can deal with them directly. In the short term there are temporary benefits to be gained from defensive coping [39]. Putting problems 'to the back of the mind' may help the individual to deal with current crisis and job demands. However, in the long term, relying solely on defensive coping efforts is likely to raise adjustment problems for the individual [53]. Long-term defensive coping may lead to physical and psychological ill health. An important issue is: at what point does defensive coping become counterproductive and stressful in itself? This remains to be found by future research.

Collective coping may be used to deal with stress and excessive work demands. Collective coping occurs within those formal and informal networks of social resources that health professionals can become involved in to mediate the impact of health care demands and stress at work [234]. House [54] viewed that these informal networks often function as 'buffers' to excessive work demands and often provide opportunities for gossiping, mutual moaning and general ventilation of feelings. Research is still in its infancy in this intricate area.

Individuals may use denial to overcome issues which are unbearable to express or talk about openly. This can be useful in distancing the doctor from the source of stress. It may also mediate in such a way that no stress is experienced by the doctor. Denial can play a positive role in achieving and maintaining detachment from stress and its sources [53] but extensive use of denial is likely to prove counterproductive in coping with stress. Denial should not interfere with successful problem solving.

In situations where doctors are dealing with death and dying patients and their relatives they may find it effective to use denial or distancing as a successful coping strategy. But continued use of denial or detachments can reduce their sensitivities to the patient's needs. In such situations regular monitoring and regular assessments of palliative coping need to be made [55]. However problem solving skills as a form of coping may be more appropriate.

It was revealed from some research that the immune system may be adversely affected by maladaptive coping strategies. In a study of women attending breast screening clinics it was found that women who keep 'emotional material' buried (particularly during periods involving stressful events such as the loss of a loved one) are significantly more at risk from breast cancer than those who are able to express their feelings, to seek help and to acknowledge the underlying stress-related events [56].

There are also some gender and situation related patterns of coping styles; males are more likely to deal with stressors by using problem-focused, and females are more likely to use emotion focused strategies [57]. Folkman and Lazarus (cited in Flanagan [57]) point out "the nature and dynamics of the situation play a role in determining the style of coping; job related stressors elicit problem focused coping, whereas health related stressors trigger emotion focused coping".

Successful coping can enable doctors to continue competently with the provision of care in such a way that does not put excessive demands on them. We will see from the studies amongst doctors (Chapter 4), that many of the coping options such as excessive alcohol consumption and drug dependency may provide temporary relief from anxiety and other more serious stress-related problems. But in the longer term, these coping strategies do not provide sustained stability or relief. Even they may increase stress and lead to more serious consequences such as cirrhosis, heart disease and suicide.

Chapter 3 – STRESS AND THE PROFESSION OF MEDICINE: Sources of Stress

In this chapter we present a model and a review of the literature illustrating the potential sources of stress. In particular, it is intended to highlight the influence of stressors inside and outside of work on the individual at work. The effect of work environment stressors are not confined to the work place but affect, in turn, an individual's family and social relations; equally, stress arising outside the workplace has an effect at work [58]. This suggests an approach to the problem of occupational stress which takes these intervening variables into account when attempting to isolate the sources and effects of stress in a specific occupational group such as GPs.

Our aim is to examine various issues in the wider context of occupational stress based upon the analysis of many different occupations over a period of twenty years or so. In any occupation there will be a large number of potential stressors. The specific stressors covered in this chapter include such factors as: intrinsic stress; work overload and time pressure; role of the GP; organisational structure; and doctors and their families (home/work interface). Also personality: Type A coronary prone behaviour pattern will be covered.

Although a review of the literature in the context of different occupations will be made, a special emphasis will be given towards reviewing literature on stressors which have particular relevance to physicians.

The stress model

In the absence of an existing conceptual framework for the specific investigation of occupational and psychosocial stressors among doctors the decision was made to adopt a simple model (see Figure 3.1). This is considered appropriate in that the factors incorporated into it were drawn from multidisciplinary fields of research, such as psychology, management sciences, medicine and sociology.

Research findings generally support the idea that the sources of stress of a particular occupation may, together with certain personality characteristics, be predictive of the manifestation of stress in the form of mental ill health, coronary heart disease (CHD), job dissatisfaction, excessive drinking and smoking, marital disharmony, etc. This can be seen from Figure 3.1, which presents a detailed proposal of a comprehensive model of occupational stress in doctors.

The model, consists of major categories of stressors: intrinsic stress; work overload; role in the organisation; organisational structure and climate; and home/work interface. These stressors are experienced by the individual doctor and the extent to which he feels impaired depends on various personal characteristics. The model also indicates major sources of occupational stress which interact with the individual doctor to result in stress outcome: job dissatisfaction; excessive drinking;

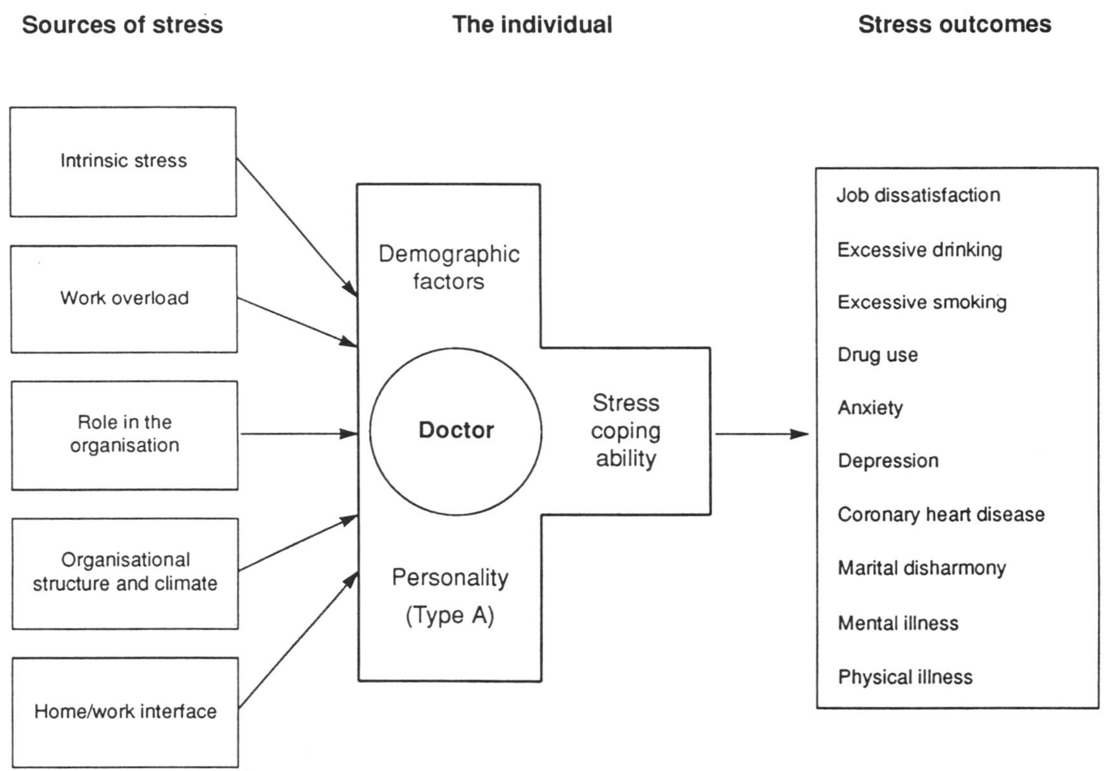

Figure 3.1. A basic theoretical model of occupational psychosocial stress in doctors

excessive smoking; drug abuse; anxiety; depression; CHD; and marital disharmony.

To date little has been done regarding the effect of occupational stress on doctors and we believe that this may be the primary cause of the condition of the 'impaired physician'. In order to understand the occupational stress syndrome in doctors several factors need to be examined. Doctors work in a chronic stress environment. Most individuals entering the health care profession have high expectations of themselves regarding their ability to help others. If they choose certain areas of medicine such as oncology, spinal trauma, and psychiatric units with chronically ill patients, they may experience a high level of stress because cures in such areas are often uncertain. In the case of GPs, they also have the responsibility of dealing with patients who are often very stressed themselves. Although GPs are self-employed people they are contracted to bear continuous responsibility 24 hours a day for their patients, which does not allow them time to relax completely.

GPs bear the responsibility for dealing with various types of stress-related problems of their patients but most of them fail to conceive that they are not exempt from the same. Over the years a myth has grown up around this profession that they are immune from the same sorts of stress-related problems as their patients. But this myth has been challenged by many researchers and evidence suggested by them carries a different view altogether. There is increased demand for improved primary health care and provision of various screening programmes. The professional demands on GPs vary widely extending from the simple cold and cough to serious physical illnesses and social problems. As the geriatric population grows rapidly their multiple disease syndrome is demanding more medical attention.

The contribution of stress, especially job related stress, to physical and psychological complaints is generally recognised by GPs. It is perhaps surprising therefore, that only recently has attention been given to the level and sources of stress in the role of the GP in the UK [59–64]. This is all the more surprising as many of the physical and psychological symptoms associated with stress show a higher incidence among GPs than other groups [65]. Problem areas can range from mild medical unfitness through general unhappiness and anxiety to more serious impairement. These include drug dependency, excessive drinking, increased smoking, divorce, psychiatric problems and suicide.

Stress as experienced by doctors

Physicians, whether they are hospital doctors or GPs, have a common duty to take care of their patients. Because of this common feature studies on 'stress in doctors' in different specialities reveal that the factors contributing to stress and its outcomes are often common to both GPs and other doctors and in this chapter studies cited referring to doctors are also applicable to GPs. In this context a study by Allibone, Oakes and Shannon [66] presents the quantitative results obtained from a postal survey concerning the major differences between hospital doctors and GPs in relation to the health and health care of physicians. The survey included only doctors who were in active medical practice in the UK, and had qualified between 1935 and 1959.

Of the 932 respondents, 361 were hospital doctors, 411 were GPs and 160 others (e.g. community physicians, academics and so on). There appeared to be very few major differences between hospital doctors and GPs in the particular age group the investigators examined, in either their medical history or their medical care.

In reported medical histories, for example, respiratory tuberculosis had occurred among hospital doctors whereas other respiratory diseases were slightly more common among GPs. This supports the view that minor upper respiratory infections are common among GPs and paediatricians, perhaps because of the known high incidences of these infections in young children. There were more diseases of the digestive track among GPs than hospital doctors. It is more difficult to generalise from the open comments made by doctors. It was found that GPs showed anxiety about the provision of locums. On the other hand, hospital doctors expressed anxiety about the need for the formal management of illness and routine medical examination. Also they showed anxiety about the danger of delay in seeking medical help, work overload, effect on family, alcohol and drugs, and privacy for doctors as patients. It was seen that more GPs delayed longer in seeking help for their illnesses than hospital doctors.

Intrinsic stress

Doctors experience stress almost everyday as an intrinsic part of their medical practice and this is unavoidable. Those who are unable to cope with such stress are likely to become 'impaired physicians'. Efficient physicians usually adapt to the stresses of medical practice and hence are able to provide improved medical care. Unfortunately in others, adaptations are often unproductive, resulting in poor quality care. This may also affect their personal and family life.

McCue [67] pointed out the stresses that he believes are intrinsic to the practice of medicine: dealing with death and suffering, sexuality, fear, problem patients and uncertainty. Linn *et al.* [68] were able to support some of these observations: having to deal with intensely emotional aspects of patients' lives, such as suffering, sexuality or death; having to deal with difficult or problem patients; meeting the needs and demands of patients; and having spontaneous home activities interrupted by work-related telephone calls. Krakowski [69] also found that the most prevalent work-related stressors for physicians were dealing with 'non-compliant and disobedient patients', and 'caring for dying patients' or those 'not responding to treatment'.

Dealing with death and suffering

Part of the work of doctors involves 'dealing with death and dying' patients where events produced feelings of inadequacy and powerlessness. The death of a patient may not only be considered as a failure of medicine or professional medical care but also taken very personally by the doctor [67].

Telling the truth about dying is a major social issue because nobody likes to talk about the realities of death. Therefore, the doctor faces the dilemma of hiding the truth from the patient but at the same time involving the family in preparing to face the inevitable outcome. It is worth noting a study by Crammond [70] in a survey of all local doctors whose names appeared in the South Australian Medical Register in which his questionnaire included items concerning the most stressful areas of clinical practice. The physicians anxieties were therapeutic failure, diagnostic difficulties, the impact of work on their family life and death of young patients.

The GP has the most ongoing contact with patients and closer involvement with the event. This makes it hard for him to reveal the terminal outcome of the disease and which ultimately causes anxiety within himself.

Glaser and Strauss [71] have provided a useful explanation which throws light upon the 'negotiations' which surround the patient/staff (nurse) interaction. It can also be applicable to patient/doctor interaction in dealing with death and suffering. This takes a number of forms which they refer to as 'the four awareness contexts'.

(1) 'Closed' – The patient does not know that he is dying and the doctor attempts to keep this from him;
(2) 'Suspicion' – The patient has an idea that he is dying and tries to confirm it but the doctor pretends;
(3) 'Mutual pretence' – Both patient and the doctor know that death is inevitable, although both pretend;
(4) 'Open' – Both patient and doctor face up to the fact that death is inevitable and act on this awareness.

Each of these prospectives will have a different effect upon the relationship between the doctor and the patient depending upon the negotiations that are necessary to sustain it. Each option presents its own problems and stressors.

'Closed' – If the patient has to be encouraged in the hope of recovery and to motivate him there must be 'conspiracy of silence'.

'Suspicion' – If the patient becomes suspicious of his true condition and tries to get information the doctor may find himself under pressure and uncertainty.

'Mutual pretence' – This may be difficult to maintain, when dependents are involved or when the patient is unwilling to face death.

'Open' – In this case the doctor and patient are no longer obliged to pretend about the prognosis and both of them move on to deal with the reality of death and stressors that this will cause.

This suggests that it is the doctor who must seek to maintain these 'negotiations', and it is likely to increase the stress attached to his job.

Cartwright *et al.* [72] found that no more than 15% of terminally ill cancer patients are told of their prognosis either by their GP or by a hospital doctor. On the contrary, almost 90% of the immediate relatives of terminally ill patients are aware of the situation and most of them learn this from the GP or hospital doctor. This may be due to the fact that doctors are often unwilling to tell patients directly that they are dying. It should be noted that although questions concerning difficulties in coping with death and suffering are often included in questionnaire survey studies, it is not reported as being a significant problem to doctors [60]. It can be suggested however, that if doctors are asked simply to report events 'dealing with death and suffering' answering such questions represent some difficulties.

Problem patients

Doctors may feel frustrated at not being able to resolve the problems of some 'problem patients'. Patients who are seen as 'uncooperative' i.e. refuse to accept all or part of the clinical regime, or refuse to accept the dependency that the sick role implies, or are very demanding or are frequent attenders to the surgery without any illness or who bring social problems, are likely to be labelled 'problem patients'. These 'problem' patients create a considerable degree of stress for doctors. It has also been suggested that recent increases in public awareness and knowledge has led to a more questioning and demanding attitude on behalf of many patients.

The amount of time spent in caring for problem patients has increased dramatically over the past three decades [67]. These patients seek medical care more often than ordinary patients. Many problem patients have some psychiatric disorder which is the basis of their frustrating interaction with doctors, but the time and energy required caring for them may deter doctors from making the psychiatric diagnosis. It is important to note that doctors are rarely taught the techniques needed for taking care of these types of patients or understanding their own feelings towards them. In Cartwright's classic studies of 1964 and 1977 [9,73] the proportion of doctors who said that they would like to spend more time with patients with psychiatric or emotional problems fell from 62% to 41%. This shows the change of attitude of the doctors. In the interview sample of 42 doctors, the authors found that all of them felt it was inappropriate for people to seek help from their doctors for non-medical and personal problems. They regarded a higher proportion of their consultations as trivial, inappropriate, or unnecessary.

The same study by Cartwright showed that the proportion of doctors who felt it appropriate for people to seek help from their GPs for problems in their family lives had fallen from 87% in 1964 to 67% in 1977. It would seem that in 1977 doctors thought that a higher proportion of their consultations were for inappropriate reasons. It was also found that the proportion of surgery consultations that they felt were for trivial, unnecessary, or inappropriate reasons rose from 24% to 38%. Therefore, 'a decrease in the proportion of doctors giving support to patients with family problems is part of their job is likely to lead to an increase in discontent among doctors'. Rankin and colleagues have suggested that GPs derive pleasure from the exercise of their technical skills [74], but what may make a particular patient a problem is not often their medical condition, but the doctor's lack of social skills.

Physical attack from the mentally ill and drug addicted patients is not uncommon [75,76]. A survey of urban GPs showed that 60 out of the 110 questioned had been attacked [77].

GPs are also uncertain about discriminating between dangerous and non-dangerous patients. Doctors reported that a substantial proportion of physical attacks occurred when on visits, and GPs are often tense when visiting 'bad areas' [78].

Uncertainty

The stress of uncertainty of the doctor lies in making serious clinical decisions on the basis of conflicting, incomplete, and untimely data. Uncertainty in consultation is inevitable but often denied [79]. The increased demand by patients for a definite diagnosis and the difficulty of the doctor to balance this with that of the cost effectiveness policies of the health care planners can make the diagnosis and treatment of even a simple sore throat into a series of uncertain decisions [67]. A simple presentation of symptoms does not always result in a straightforward diagnosis. There remains a remote possibility of a sinister pathology for which the doctor takes the gamble to exclude the odds but in turn creates stress for himself. Taking this kind of brave decision may alleviate his fears temporarily but exposure of falsehood may cause problems with communication between the doctor and the patient, and may create moral and emotional problems for the doctor. On the other hand doctors may choose thorough investigations on each and every trivial illness to arrive at a diagnosis in order to avoid stress but such a policy will not be cost effective for the health service and has little clinical benefits.

Another problem of 'uncertainty' is the content of the day's work. Rankin *et al.* [74] have examined the factors associated with self-reported negative mood changes in GPs. Just over half of these changes were associated with a combination of 'hassle' (unexpected demands, intrusions and delays) and 'time pressure'. Interruptions of one kind or another make the GP uncertain about his days plan which ultimately pressurise him.

Sexuality

An important aspect of the doctor–patient relationship seldom talked about is the physical one. The doctor is often required to conduct intimate examinations of patients. He may have ambivalent feelings because of his civilized desire to respect the modesty of the patient and avoid the anxiety of physical nakedness. Students and interns are most vulnerable to the stresses of embarrassment [80].

Work overload and time pressure

Both qualitative (too difficult) and quantitative (too much to do) work overload are potential stressors to GPs. Increased demand by the patients on the GPs to provide comprehensive and continuing care imposes increasing stress on them. The first systematic survey on patients and GPs was carried out by Cartwright in 1964 [73]. The lay respondents in her survey commented, 'Doctors today are overworked. If they had fewer patients they could give them more time'. It can be hypothesized that GPs feel overloaded with work. Being a self-employed group of professionals they have to consider the administrative aspect of running their practice whilst at the same time taking care of patients and keeping pace with medical advancement. The most frequently acknowledged stressor was lack of time [81,82]. In 1977 Cartwright found that 20% of GPs were pressurised for time [83]. The GPs mentioned: 'Not enough time ever to do one's work adequately and still have time to live a normal family life' [9]. When working faster, doctors deal less adequately with psychosocial problems, and pressure of time also affects judgement in other areas [82].

A study of 180 physicians who were alumni of the Case Western Reserve School of Medicine reported that the sources of dissatisfaction in the lives of these physicians were not having personal free time, being on call and carrying a heavy workload [84]. Mechanic [85] found that time factors were a major source of dissatisfaction for physicians in primary care settings. Linn *et al.* [68] in their physician sample of 221 on the University College of Los Angeles faculty found that time pressure of various kinds were the most frequently endorsed sources of physician distress. Mawardi [84] viewed that in the USA private practitioners rated time related stresses as their greatest dissatisfaction. The doctors felt that the demands of the workload and continuous on call responsibility leaves very little personal time. It is obvious that work overload is one of the main sources of stress that GPs identify in themselves. Therefore it is perhaps worth noting some studies which are related to nature of work, volume of work and timetable of work in general practice.

McDonald and McLean [86] reported that the average working week in south east Scotland was 39 hours (with a range of 26–53 hours) and that 76 hours were spent on call (with a range of 37–102 hours). Richardson *et al.* [87] found that in a typical week the average GP was consulted on 180 occasions. Howie [88] reported that consultation rates have been falling over the last 15 years or so; also home visiting rates are decreasing as well (55 visits per week reported in the 1970s [86]; 40 visits per week per doctor in 1980 [89]. Even though consultation rates and home visits have fallen there are other aspects of the GPs job which contribute to their work overload. It was found, for example, that there were 1.7 indirect consultation per patients per year [88] which contribute substantially to workload and stress of the GP. Finishing surgery or home visits does not mean the end of the days work. There are referrals to be made, problems arising from consultation to be sorted out (such as arrangements of transport for patients to attend the outpatients department) and delegation of responsibilities to paramedical staff has to be detailed also.

Night work is another source of work overload for the GP. For those GPs who provide out-of-hours cover, the loss and disruption of sleep may be similar to the stress associated with long working hours or shift work. General practitioners who provide maternity care, single handed rural GPs, and those who cover their practices during the night time, without using deputising service, are bound to have disturbed sleep. Disturbed sleep patterns cán cause deterioration in health and well being in the GP, which may in turn exacerbate other factors such as interpersonal relationship at work and at home, efficiency and judgement.

The role of the GP

An individual's role at work has been isolated as a main source of occupational stress, involving role ambiguity (lack of clarity about one's job) and role conflict (conflicting job demands), as well as responsibility for people and conflicts stemming from organisational boundaries. It has been suggested that the organisational stressors stemming from role ambiguity and role conflict can result in such stress related illness as coronary heart disease [90].

Role ambiguity

Role ambiguity results when the individual does not have adequate information about his work role and the behaviour that is expected. Kahn *et al.* [91] found that men who suffered from role ambiguity experienced lower job satisfaction, high job related tension, greater futility and lower self confidence.

A GP may be faced with a difficult situation (like managing a cancer patient), and find it extremely difficult to reveal the diagnosis because it may unproductively upset the patient. On the other hand, withholding the true diagnosis is depriving the patient of knowing his condition. This is an example of role ambiguity in a profession where there is a lack of clarity about one's job. This situation is a source of extreme pressure on the GP where he experiences stress and anxiety. In this case the conflict is internal and results from feelings of uncertainty caused by unclear responsibilities.

Role conflict

Kahn *et al.* [91] have defined role conflict as "the simultaneous occurrence of two or more sets of pressures such that compliance with one would make more difficult compliance with other". According to Cooper and Marshall [58], role conflict exists when an individual in his environment is torn by conflicting job demands; doing things that he does not really want to do or does not believe are part of his job. Kahn *et al.* [91] found that men who suffered more role conflict had lower job satisfaction and higher job related tension.

In general practice the element of practice administration is an additional responsibility on top of clinical practice. There is an increased feeling amongst the new generation of GPs that they would function more efficiently without this element of practice administration which is creating conflicting job demands and therefore contributing to stress. On top of this the new contract proposes that GPs handle their own budgets, in which case they not only have to be clinicians but also accountants as well; unless they are careful in spending, they may have to face penalties.

A useful model (see Figure 3.2) which locates the sources of stress within general practice illustrates the role of the GP. Basically four 'sets of expectations' in the GPs role can be identified. Three of these arise from external sources and one is internal to the individual.

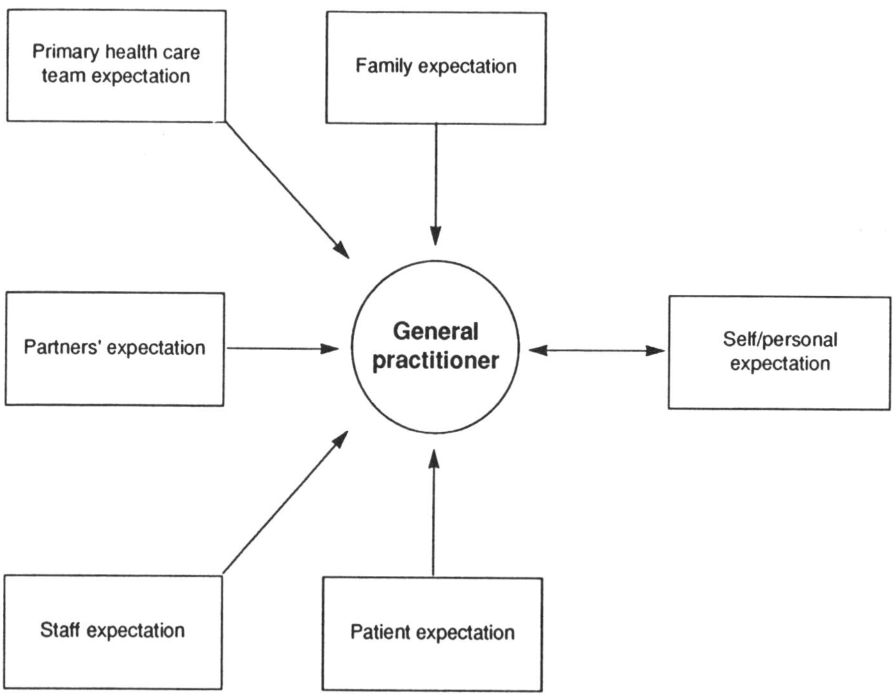

Figure 3.2. The central role of the GP

Stress can arise from:

1. Organisational expectations (partners' expectations, primary health care team's expectations, staff expectations, FHSA expectations, professional expectations).
2. Patient expectations.
3. Family expectations.
4. Personal/self expectations.

When the expectations from these four sources are consistent and balanced then the role is clearly defined for the GP. When two or more sources of expectations clash then role conflict is likely to result.

1. Organisational expectations

From a professional point of view the GP holds the value of patient care as central to his role yet the organisational expectation is different. He is expected to have cordial relationship with his staff, members of primary health care team and his partners in order to function efficiently and satisfactorily. The primary health care team includes district nurse, health visitor, social worker, community psychiatric nurse, community midwife, chiropodist and even pharmacist. Within such a dynamic situation the GP may find himself involved in an interdependent relationship with a perplexing variety of specialisms. Each of these relationships will involve a set of expectations concerning his role and how he should act.

The changing responsibilities and relationships with the development of primary health care teams might be stressful for the GP [92,93]. Discussing patient care with partners and the primary health care team is often seen as unproductive by some GPs in the absence of any definitive guidelines.

Large numbers of GPs are in group practices where they are more likely to come into conflict with their partners on various matters. The problem may be related to the differences in expectations of each other. Younger GPs or new principals may find the attitudes of senior partners to be totally different from their own. They may feel that senior colleagues are too rigid in accepting new and innovative ideas. Therefore, they may get frustrated and dissatisfied.

It is uncommon to see mid-career change in general practice. General practitioners reach their financial peak during their early 30's. In the non-hierarchical structure of general practice, partnership are meant for an indefinite period. In circumstances when an established GP applies for a practice vacancy elsewhere, suspicions may arise amongst the partners. In many cases a GP may feel as if he has nowhere to go and hence puts up with role conflict. Role conflict can also occur when a senior partner or partners in a group practice want a junior partner to do something that he does not like or want to do or conversely when younger partners with new and innovative ideas pressurise senior partners.

2. Patient expectations

Role conflict occurs as the GP attempts to satisfy a number of incompatible demands arising from different patients' expectations of his role.

Patients' expectations today have risen so high that some GPs find it extremely difficult to cope. Many GPs feel that they are being used. One GP commented:

"It is unfair that GPs' out-of-hours work begins at 11 pm when most other workers finish at 5 pm every day. The basic practice allowance and supplementary practice allowance practically buys a doctor's service and his destiny. This money forces the doctor to be on call every evening and night of the year, including bank holidays, and thereby deprives him of his family and social life, hence divorce and suicide rates are increasing among doctors." [94]

3. *Family expectations*

Work is only one aspect of the total life activity for any individual. Every individual has many roles to play in society and in the family. A GP may have the role of husband or wife, father or mother, son or daughter, a member of a social or political group, etc. When the demands of work and non-work roles become incompatible the GP faces conflict as to which to give priority.

An episode of illness in the family can create a role conflict in the doctor/father or doctor/mother if there is a demand for involvement. There is the conflict between what the doctor father and/or mother are actually doing and what the family expects them to do, which causes identity dilemmas. In this case the doctor wishes to treat his family but at the same time he is worried in case anything goes wrong. He may get confused whether he should play the role as the parent or behave like a doctor. Even in a simple and natural event such as the birth of a baby it can be difficult where the mother needs her husband to be wholly husband, the doctor husband may not be able to forget his professional role – in checking the actions of a doctor and nurses [141].

In the case of women doctors, role conflict seems to be more pronounced. Besides her professional duty, the husband may still expect his working doctor wife to carry out the traditional household duties. Ducker [95] found that while a high level of commitment to either profession or family reduced role conflict, high commitment to both produced severe conflict. Therefore, this type of home/work conflict causes a great deal of stress to many GPs.

4. *Personal/self expectation*

We believe that many of the unrealistic expectations are internalised by the profession itself, due largely to the acceptance of society's stereotyping and through the process of professional socialisation. Socialisation of the doctor with professional colleagues may produce unreasonable and irrational expectations.

The GP recognises the value given to him by the society as a 'Godly person' who can significantly influence patients' lives. Because of this professional myth the GP is reluctant to come down to the level of a patient when he has an illness or problem. Although many studies reveal the existence of excessive alcohol consumption, drug abuse and suicide (discussed in the next chapter) within the medical profession the individual does not seek help. Besides, his partners and colleagues do not expect him to become ill.

Responsibility for people

'Responsibility' has been identified as a potential stressor associated with one's role in the organisation. Both responsibility for people and responsibility for things have been identified as stressors but responsibility for people is more likely to be a stressor than responsibility for things. Many authors acknowledged that responsibility for people is significantly more likely to lead to coronary heart disease (CHD) than responsibility for things [96,97]. French and Caplan [97], found that responsibility for people was related to serum cholesterol levels, diastolic blood pressure and heavy smoking.

Increased responsibility for people means that the individual has to spend more time interacting with others, attending meetings, working alone and, in consequence, more time in trying to meet deadline pressures and schedules [97]. Cobb and Rose [98] found that hypertension among air traffic controllers was four times higher than it was in the control group (second class airmen). The incidence of hypertension was higher still for those air traffic controllers working in high density traffic towers. Peptic ulcers was twice as frequent in the air traffic controllers and there was a suggestion that diabetes was more common. Cobb and Rose [98] ascribe the results to "the close attention involved and the heavy responsibility the individual shoulders with respect to other people's lives" (i.e. responsibility for people).

General practitioners carry a great deal of responsibility for other people where wrong decisions made by them may lead to the exacerbation of the disease or even death of the patient. Increasing responsibility for people leading to increasing stress makes GPs susceptible to many stress related diseases. Data on peptic ulcer disease have shown a great excess of ulcers among physicians [99]. If we compare within the profession it is evident that anaesthesiologists and GPs take more death responsibility than dermatologists and pathologists. Russek and Sohen [100], showed that anaesthesiologists and GPs reported two to three times as much CHD as dermatologists. Without comparable incidence and mortality information, such prevalent differences may be misleading. Nevertheless, according to a British study of doctors [65], the incidence of and mortality from, myocardial infarcts is about twice as high in GPs aged 40 to 60 as in other members of the profession of comparable age. In general then one must suspect that mortality rate for CHD is higher in doctors in general. The higher mortality rate due to CHD may be coincidental with frequency of type A personality among physicians [101] who in general represent a sizeable population of compulsive personalities when compared with other professions. Type A personality is discussed in a later part of this chapter.

Organisational structure and climate

Another potential source of stress for the doctor arises from the organisation itself – its structure and climate, which can make working life either satisfactory or stressful: such as little or no participation in the decision making process, lack of effective consultation and restrictions in behaviour (e.g. budgets) [58].

One of the major issues here is employee participation in the work place. Organisations differ in the extent in which they allow and encourage participation in decision making and this difference in approach may show in the health of employees. French and Caplan [97] found that opportunity for participation in decision making produced significantly greater job satisfaction, higher feelings of self esteem and lower job related feelings of threat. In a national sample survey Margolis, Kroes and Quinn [102] found non-participation at work was a consistent and significant predictor of strain and job-related stress. It was found to be related to health risk factors, including overall poor physical health, escapist drinking, depressed mood, low self esteem, low life satisfaction, low job satisfaction, low motivation to work, intention to leave jobs and absenteeism from work. Participation in decision making processes on the part of the individual may help to increase his 'investment' in the organisation, create a sense of belonging and improve communication channels within the organisation.

Nowadays partnerships are the norm in British general practice. For effective functioning it is important that there is close cooperation, communication and participation amongst the partners. Some group practices hold regular meetings for partners to be present to discuss matters but some do not meet as a group for mutual support, problem solving or policy making. Even though meetings are held at regular intervals, the senior partners often have greater influence while the junior partners are sometimes neglected. In other cases the practice managers are not even invited to sit in the practice meetings. There remains a gap between the policy making by the partners and the role of the practice manager whose responsibility is to manage the staff. Therefore, there is no direct contact between the doctors and ancillary staff. Sometimes without putting an effort to maintain the atmosphere of cooperation GPs create, confusion and chaos within the practice set up.

It has been claimed that reductions in hospital services are imposing an increasing strain on GPs, which they can no longer be expected to absorb. One Buckinghamshire GP said that undercutting of hospital services inevitably rebounded on primary care, which already deals with 90% of cases. 'The reality is that GPs are being asked to do more and more with less and less resources and that is a strain which we can't and shouldn't have to take'.

Another restriction on GPs behaviour is the problem of staff appointment. GPs surgeries cannot be seen as a homogeneous category. They are varied in structure, purpose, size and location. Some doctors practice in purpose built health centres provided by the Area Health Authority, and others in their own premises (some purpose built and others converted). Many practices do require additional staff in order to keep the records up-to-date and office work efficient. There is a severe restriction from the government which allows only two full time secretaries per doctor, for the purpose of ancillary staff pay reimbursement. This restriction limits GPs' liberty in employing more staff.

Doctors and their families

It is the nature of most professions that the boundary between work and non-work is often indistinct and blurred, and inevitably there will be some degree of 'overflow' in both directions. Although stress is predominantly work-related, sufferers get caught in a vicious circle of neglecting the family life for which stress at work also increases. Research into occupational stress and family life has presented evidences that excessive involvement of husbands and wives in demanding occupational roles, can have an adverse effect on the family [103–106]. Most GPs complained that general practice seriously conflicted with family life [77].

A number of writers [106,107] give importance to wives' behaviour and attitudes in bettering or reducing the effect of stress on the family. For example, Burke *et al.* [108] examined the compatability of 190 husband–wife pairs (husbands with either accountants or engineers) and their impact on stress management. They found that the more compatible were the wives and husbands, the greater was the likelihood of coping with stress-related problems at work and at home. Doctors are not different from these occupational groups in relation to their family and social life. Marriages and sexual relationships are often unsatisfactory for doctors [84,109,110], although divorce may be no more common than in the general population [111,112].

The doctor's wife

Almost all of the significant literature available on married doctors considers the traditional male–doctor female–wife partnership and there are very few studies examining female doctors and male husbands or indeed other types of stable relationships.

Kennie's survey [114] on doctors' wives showed that they are the most neglected patients and are often not taken notice of before becoming seriously ill. Other studies suggest that doctors' wives perhaps suffer more due to the attitudes of doctors and nurses who consider them differently to other patients in terms of complications or poor outcomes [115,116]. Dearlove [115] carried out a study on a group of doctors and their pregnant wives, comparing them with two control groups of similar social class for obstetric, paediatric and psychiatric complications. The proportion of minor psychiatric problems was significantly different between the two groups but there was no difference when paediatric and obstetric outcomes were compared in spite of the preferential care that the experimental group received. Even though problems were observed by the medical staff they were hesitant in passing on the information once they had become aware of the status of the patient. The authors put it thus: ". . . her husband expects her to behave very differently from his own patients and consequently she is effectively ignored by everyone dealing with her emotional care".

Sakinofsky's [117] Canadian study found that doctors' wives were four times more likely to commit suicide than other women. Also there is evidence from psychiatrists to show that doctors' wives do suffer from emotional stress [113,118,119] and this is harmful. When there is a marital problem, denial may take the form of (a) writing a prescription for his wife or sending her to a psychiatrist, (b) withdrawal into longer hours at the office, or (c) passive and condescending tolerance of her angry outbursts [113].

Bird [120] pointed out some danger signals in the medical marriage. These include when the physician's wife "becomes painfully disillusioned or painfully deceived when she discovers that what she had perceived as strength in her strong, unafraid, efficient and unemotional husband really represents emotional control and detachment". He describes how the physician responds to his wife's anger in an emotionally detached way. The defences used here are denial and isolation of affect which is also used as a defence mechanism in medical practice. This emotional distance of the physician enhances his wife's anger and the response pattern by the physician is repeated. He then describes that the doctors are "not the world's best lovers"; their commitment to medicine and their patients do not "place a high premium on the romantic arts".

Nelson [113] quotes a study (by Harrison: personal communication) on doctors' wives in which the finding was that 95% of sample questioned 'felt neglected'. She said 'the doctor's practice seems as a demanding mistress who always wins. Physicians can use the demands of their practice to shield themselves from the demands of wife and family'. Psychiatric breakdown in doctors' children is significantly high, and the rate of suicide amongst doctors' wives is five times higher than that amongst the wives of architects and accountants [121].

Miles, Krell and Lin [122] studied 20 physician's wives who had been inpatients in British Colombia and found the following: 90% had a primary diagnosis of depression, 95% had personality disorders of hysterical and passive aggressive types, 90% had a history of suicidal ideation or attempts, and 54% had drug and/or alcohol problems.

Women doctors

The number of married working women has increased substantially in the UK. Twenty-five years ago only 25% of working women were married; by 1980 this had increased to 60% [123]. Involvement in both work and the family is likely to be stressful for the female physician. Today, 70% of married women work and over 41% of women with a child under five years of age are in employment, compared with 24% in 1983 [124]. Despite working full-time, women are often expected to meet domestic commitments. There is some evidence that conflicting demands from work and family can be stressful. Cooper [125] found that more and more married women are either divorcing, limiting their family size, or coping with both worlds at the expense of their physical and psychological health.

Rose and Roscow [126] found that the divorce rate for female doctors is higher than the general population. The ratio of divorces for female doctors compared with male doctors is 3 to 2. More female doctors are single than male doctors. The percentage for female doctors is 31% and for male doctors 8%.

The effects of stress in female doctors are reflected in the four-fold increased risk of suicide compared to other social class [127] and the findings that 46% of a sample of women house officers fulfilled the criteria for clinical depression [128].

It should be noted that three sources of stress are reported to be more common in women: external prejudice, fragmentation and normative value conflicts [83,95,129,130]. Cartwright [131] found that women doctors of Japanese ancestry educated in the late 1960s and early 1970s were more stressed. These women doctors suffered from sex role inadequacy in their own culture which raised the question of assertiveness and dominance in women. Although such behaviour was expected by the profession it offered little support. Hence anxiety and career dissatisfactions were seen amongst these career women.

The second major source of stress is fragmentation [131] or role strain [132]. Role strain occurs when there are two or more significant role obligations. This strain is a product of conflict between occupational and traditional sex roles for women. Therefore women doctors with the role of wife, mother as well as physician suffer from fragmentation.

The third major source of stress stems from internal normative value conflict [133]. Each role (role of woman and role of doctor) demands different direction and roles may clash on an unconscious level. Guilt, worry, as well as identity dilemmas, can be emotional consequences of feelings of failure at both roles. The desire to satisfy both the roles may lead to exhaustion.

Heins *et al.* [134] found that women doctors spend 90% as much time in medical practice as men doctors while tending to assume direct responsibility for home and family and hence they have the added burden of trying to balance the demands imposed by both sides. Nadelson and Notman [129] point out that women are traditionally expected to assume direct responsibility for their own parents and husbands which is an added source of stress during the medical career. It was found that women doctors were particularly stressed by the pressures and desires to be with their children and other dual career issues (e.g. financial burden of providing good household help) [135]. As a result of these stresses, more women are working part time employment and taking salaried positions than men [129,134,136,137]; they are also more likely to interrupt practice and training [83,138]. It was also found that women are more likely than men to enter a specialty which is not their first choice [139] and many more women than men fail to achieve their desired status in general practice (i.e. GP principal) [140].

The cause of stress in the doctors' family have been analysed by several doctors' wives [113,141,142], but these papers have been anecdotal, and little quantitative research appears to have been done in this area.

Personality: behaviour patterns

The interactive view of stress is that situations are not inherently stressful. The psychological, physiological or/and behavioural consequence of organisational stressors are the product of the particular situation, and the individual with his specific personality, behaviour pattern and life circumstances. Therefore different individuals will react differently to the same environment. Some individuals are better able to cope with the stressors at work than others; they adapt their behaviour in a way that meets the environmental challenge. On the other hand, some individuals are psychologically predisposed to stress: they are unable to cope or adapt to the stress provoking situations. The area of study receiving most attention appears to be 'personality differences' between high and low stressed individuals.

Personality in doctors

Doctors have often been described as compulsive and achievement oriented. This compulsiveness may be increased during the training period. It was observed by Krakowski [69] that 100% of physicians ($n = 100$) who were polled randomly declared themselves 'compulsive personalities'. The criteria on which he assessed the physician subjects were: restricted ability to warm and tender emotions, perfectionism, insistence that others submit to one's way of doing things, excessive devotion to work and productivity to the exclusion of pleasure and the value of interpersonal relationships and indecisiveness. It was found that 80% of his sample met three of the five and 20% met four out of five of the above criteria. Nelson [113] describes the physician as an 'ought-to' person who takes pride in overproduction and often has a pathologically overdeveloped ability to postpone pleasure. His life pattern has been characterised by the delay of personal satisfaction.

Gabbard [143] observed physician's compulsiveness based on the observations of those who attended the Menninger Foundation's sponsored workshop for physicians in Colorado. According to Gabbard [143] physicians' compulsiveness consists of doubt, guilt feelings, and an exaggerated sense of responsibility. Physicians with certain personality characteristics may have chosen medicine as a career and their compulsiveness is magnified during their training. Gabbard suggests the "grand paradox: compulsiveness and excessive conscientiousness are character traits that are socially valuable but personally expensive. Society's meat is the physician's poison". He further portrays the maladaptive aspects of compulsive traits which include: "difficulty in relaxing, reluctance to take vacations from work, problems in allocating time to family, an inappropriate and excessive sense of responsibility for things beyond one's control, chronic feelings of 'not being enough', difficulty in setting limits, hypertrophied guilt feelings that interfere with a healthy pursuit of pleasure, and the confusion of selfishness with healthy self-interest".

The resistance of the doctor to seeking help has been observed by many authors. The physician does not ask for help and he thinks that he should be autonomous, self-sufficient and self-controlled. Actually, he has difficulty in asking for help for himself when he is under stress. The equating of psychiatric symptoms with a sign of weakness has been a common finding. In addition, acknowledging psychiatric symptoms as part of an illness would challenge a physician's sense of omniscience, omnipotence and invulnerability. As Robinowitz [144] expresses, "Physicians may use their knowledge and skills to defend themselves against their own anxiety about strength, both integrity and dangers of illness and health".

It can be suggested that physicians may be unaware of their stress problems. Often they are connected to occupational demands [111]. Generally physicians adopt a tough-minded approach to human problems, dislike expression of emotion and introspection [145]. They are often defensively locked into self-important, authoritarian professional roles [67].

Type A coronary prone behaviour

The major research approach to individual stress differences began with the work of Friedman and Rosenman [101,146,147] in the early 1960s and developed later establishing a relationship between certain behavioural patterns and the prevalence of CHD. These behavioural patterns were later referred to as 'coronary prone behaviour pattern type A' (high risk of CHD), and were distinguished from 'Type B' (low risk of CHD).

Type A behaviour is recognisable in individuals who display aggressiveness, feelings of being under the challenge of responsibility, haste, extreme competitiveness, strive for achievement, impatient, restlessness, hyperalertness, explosiveness of speech, tenseness of facial muscles, excessive drive and distinct sense of time urgency [148]. The most significant trait of the type A man is his ceaseless sense of time urgency or 'hurry sickness'. The type A man persistently strives to accomplish too much or participate in too many events in the amount of time he assigns for these purposes. It is the type A man's contentious struggle with time, that Friedman and Rosenman [148] believe so frequently leads to his early death from CHD. It has been suggested by Jenkins [149] that individuals having the type A behavioural pattern were "often so deeply involved and committed to their work that other aspects of their lives were relatively neglected".

Type B individuals are characterised by Jenkins *et al.* [150] as being more relaxed and easy going, rarely becoming impatient; not easily irritated, working steadily without a feeling of being driven by time pressure, and speaking in a slower and more modulated manner. Rosenman, Friedman and Straus [101] suggest that this dichotomy is not a sharp division as "the subject with behaviour pattern A simply exhibits to an enhanced and sometimes excessive degree and certain traits which are variously present in subject with pattern B but to a lesser degree. Thus, the elevation of the body temperature or blood pressure . . . which normally are exhibited by all subjects".

In early studies, individuals were designated as type A or type B on the basis of clinical judgements of doctors and psychologists or peer ratings. The criticism of these early studies were that they were retrospective in nature, but this methodological weakness was overcome in the classic Western Collaborative Group Study in the mid-sixties [101,146]. This was a prospective study of over 34,000 men, which began in 1959 and continued over the years to produce data of an epidemiological, pathological and biochemical nature, relating aggressive emotion with a high risk of getting CHD [151]. This study also confirmed the importance of such factors as family history of CHD, elevated systolic and diastolic blood pressures, cigarette smoking, level of education and raised serum levels of cholesterol, beta lipoproteins and natural fat.

The original study began by classifying individuals as type A or type B on the basis of structured interviews: none had a prior record of heart disease. Results of follow-up investigations at regular intervals have confirmed type A behaviour pattern as a precursor of CHD, independent of the standard risk factors, such as: blood pressure, age, serum lipids, cigarette smoking, age, and parental history of CHD [146,152]. Those judged to be type A at the outset of the study had twice the rate of clinical coronary diseases, were five times as likely to get a second myocardial infarction and had twice the rate of fatal heart attacks experienced by the type B subjects at the eight-and-a-half year follow-up investigation. Many other studies have since supported roughly the same findings [153–156].

The issue of 'self selection' into jobs that require a greater exposure to stressors needs to be considered in that persons with a particular personality and behaviour characteristics might pursue a certain type of work environment. For example, McMichael [157] suggests that the nature of type A behavioural traits may provoke some degree of self-selection, by those who possess them, into occupations which involve greater exposure to stressors. This notion is supported by the findings of Caplan *et al.* [155]. House [158] has suggested that the aggressive, ambitious and competitive elements of type A behaviour may be exhibited as a status seeking or intrinsic work motivation, i.e. desire for status, money, recognition etc. and that this may lead to self-selection into occupations where the opportunity to satisfy such motivations is greatest.

It may be that type A individuals are more prone to perceive stress in an exaggerated fashion [159]. This would appear to be instinctively relevant to studies of stress in GPs. It can be suggested that GPs with type A personalities may plan their working day in a different way to those GPs of type B personality. They may subjectively perceive the workload by their style of behaviour and may create their own stress. This may be self-imposed rather than due to the actual job requirement. The GPs with type A personalities may be inclined to take more responsibility, for example, in surgery administration and NHS commitments and less responsibility for family life. Even after perceiving more stressors they may self-record low levels of strain as part of denial or suppression.

It remains to be seen whether the GPs were of type A personality before entering into general practice or whether they develop or intensify such personality after entering into the profession. Rosenman [160] strongly proposed that many people do not possess type A characteristics when they enter an occupation but increased time pressures, demands for speed and conscientiousness required by the job can convert a relaxed type B into a type A.

Dembrowski *et al.* [161] consider that ". . . type A subjects are more aggressive, more time urgent, more impatient and more hard driving than type B when appropriate environmental challenges are made salient" and indicate that this point underlines the importance of the environment in eliciting type A behaviour.

Glass *et al.* [162] demonstrated the importance of the competitive nature of the challenge task in determining both cardiovascular and catecholamine stress responses. Type A and type B subjects played a competitive electronic game under two conditions i.e harassment versus no harassment condition. It was found that during the harassment condition, that type A subjects showed a greater increase in heart rate, systolic blood pressure and plasma epinephrine than did type B subjects but not in the non-harassment condition. This study confirms that type A individuals do not respond to all situations as relevant stressors, and that it is only when the properties of the stressor situation are perceived as such that the type A is so challenged that cardiovascular responses are pronounced. These responses may contribute to the higher relative risk of CHD that is associated with the type A behaviour pattern. In general practice, Porter, Howie and Levinson [59] found that extreme type A personalities are more likely to report feelings of stress than extreme type B personalities. However, the authors warn that considerable caution should be taken, because only 4 out of the 15 doctors fell into these categories.

Much less data on type A behaviour in employed women is available than is the case for employed men. Haynes and Feinleib [163] provide eight year data from the longitudinal Framingham heart study of 1317 subjects (580 men, 350 housewives and 387 working women) which indicates that, although working women in general did not have a significantly higher incidence of CHD than housewives and their CHD rates were lower than CHD rates for men, the CHD rates in married working women showed a substantial increase over rates for single working women. Further analysis showed that for working women the incidence for CHD rose as the number of children increased but this was not the case for housewives. Research shows that in women, as in men, there is a strong association between type A behaviour patterns and the onset of CHD [146,164]. Friedman and Rosenman [148] found even higher levels of serum cholesterol in type A women than in type A men. On the basis of the Framingham study it appears that higher scoring type A working women are twice as likely to develop CHD as type A men. Cooper and Davidson [165] suggest that one possible reason for this increased incidence is that working women are often expected to simultaneously combine the roles of housemaker and career person simultaneously.

Davidson and Cooper [166] studied 135 senior female executives and found that their sample contained over twice the proportion of the most extreme type A individuals, who are most often at risk in terms of stress-related illness. Therefore, one might suggest that in order for women to be successful, they need to be more type A individuals. Similarly, women in general practice may have a type A personality or may have to develop such a personality to be successful in a male-dominated occupation.

French and Caplan [97], reviewing the evidence of psychosocial factors in heart disease, suggest that "such a wealth of findings makes it hard to ignore type A as a relevant syndrome". Stress research needs to take into account the active interaction between environment and the person and the importance of type A behaviour pattern. Cooper and Marshall [58], emphasizing the importance of personality traits as an intervening variable in the stress equation, conclude: "it can be seen therefore that psychometric and behavioural data on individual differences play a crucial role in the person–environment fit paradigm and ultimately in the manifestation of stress-related disease".

Chapter 4 – STRESS AND THE PROFESSION OF MEDICINE: Stress Outcomes

When an individual experiences stress from either an organisational or an extra organisational source, this will manifest itself in stress outcomes specific to the individual. Some individuals may suffer from physical and/or psychiatric symptoms of ill health, while others may manifest the stress in behavioural terms, through excessive drinking, drug abuse and/or increased smoking. In this context we concentrate firstly on physical illness.

Physical illness

A limited number of studies have focussed on those physical illnesses believed to be stress-related, such as peptic ulcer and respiratory diseases but these have not been researched as thoroughly in respect to job stressors as coronary heart disease (CHD). Thus, here we concentrate mainly on CHD.

Over the last 25–30 years stress has been linked with CHD. An American Heart Association report in 1976 estimated that the annual cost of cardiovascular disease to be $26.7 billion [169]. The British Heart Foundation estimates that 180,000 people a year die from heart disease in England and Wales and this accounts for 70 million working days lost each year to industry and commerce [170]. In England and Wales the death rate due to CHD in men doubled between 1956 and 1973, and has increased much more rapidly in younger than in older age ranges. By 1973, 41% of all deaths in the age range 25–44 were due to cardiovascular diseases [169].

There is statistical evidence suggesting that occupational stress is a causal factor in such stress-related diseases as CHD [41]. Carruthers [151] suggests that it is those occupational stressors which encourage the emotions of anger, frustration and aggression which may contribute significantly to CHD. There are also a number of studies which support the proposition that the risk of CHD rises with occupational level [96,175–178].

Nevertheless, the idea that CHD is found predominantly among white collar and professional workers has been challenged by Cooper. He reviewed British and American statistics on the incidence of death due to ischaemic heart disease in different types of occupations [169]. The frequencies of death due to ischaemic heart disease increased as one moved from white collar and professional jobs down to the unskilled level. In his review of studies on work stress [155], Cooper illustrates that the incidence of ill health was greater for blue collar workers than white collar workers. In addition, nervous strain at work was reported by a higher proportion of white collar and professional workers than that of skilled and unskilled manual workers. Thus, Cooper [169] interprets that "these results may indicate only that white collar and professional groups differ from blue collar occupations in their reactions to stress, that is, that the former reflect the pressures of work in mental illness whereas the latter do so in physical symptoms and illness".

Retrospective case control studies have shown a significant association between CHD and long working hours under stress [179,180] and professional difficulties in the past [181,182]. Prospective studies have shown the relationship between financial problems or non-specific stress and the incidence of angina [183–185] but not to myocardial infarction [185,186]. Some other studies have found a significant correlation between workload or tension at work with the incidence of myocardial infarction [187,188].

In another retrospective study, Kittel *et al.* [189] observed a significant relation between excess of CHD incidence and a job stress score. In a prospective study Sobolski *et al.* [190] found a significant relation between the job stress score and angina pectoris but not with ECG modifications suggestive of CHD.

Most studies reported rely heavily on correlational data for their conclusions. Therefore, the inferences about causality which can be drawn are limited. Correlational analysis also fails to point out the role of intervening variables. So, the influence of the natural history of CHD in those already affected needs to be considered. The incidence of CHD may be coincidental with greater frequency of personality type A among doctors.

Physical illness among doctors

It might be expected that doctors suffer more illness than the general population, because of excessive work pressure, scarcity of free time, long hours of work, irregular meals, disturbed nights or interrupted evenings and weekends, and close contact with diseases.

In the period immediately after the second world war doctors were almost twice as likely as the general population to develop a myocardial infarction [65]. In 1976, Doll and Peto found that deaths from heart disease had been declining in British doctors, and doctors under 54 years were less likely to die of ischaemic heart disease and myocardial degeneration than the general population.

In the USA death from heart disease has been more common amongst doctors than in the control population [191,192]. For example, Dublin and Spiegelman [193] showed that the rate of cardiovascular disorders was 1.8 higher than that of the general population. There may be, however, differences between those in different branches of the profession. Anaesthesiologists and GPs reported two to three times the levels of CHD of dermatologists [112]. Morris *et al.* [65] also found that GPs were twice as likely as other British doctors to develop myocardial infarct.

By analysing the statistical data published by the Registrar General in Occupational Mortality it can be verified whether doctors have an overall life expectancy different from that of the general population. These use the Standard Mortality Ratio (SMR) as a measure of risk. SMR is the ratio of observed deaths in a population divided by those expected from the national death rates, standardised for age and sex, and multiplied by 100. The figures [194] showed that overall, doctors have a standard mortality ratio of 81 – that is, in 1978 they were 19% better off than the general population. American studies have also showed similar conclusions [192,195]. Everson and Fraumeni [196] reported a similar result in expected deaths among medical students and young doctors. Dublin and Spiegelman [191,193] reported that in the years 1938–1942 doctors in general had almost the same longevity and mortality as the general population. Goodman [197] showed that in the years 1969–1973 during which the medical population in the USA reached almost 345,000, doctors' deaths averaged about 3800 annually. When doctors were compared with the US white population of the same age and sex, doctors death rates were lower than expected for white males and females. The findings of 1969–1973 compared with those of 1938–1942 [191,193] revealed that the working life expectancy of doctors was higher.

The improved survival of doctors may be attributed to their higher socio-economic status and greater chances to seek treatment promptly [195] and especially access to specialised medical treatment. Their knowledge of health risks may also contribute to improve survival rate. Doll and Peto [198] demonstrated the beneficial effects achieved by doctors due to decreased smoking. The cigarette consumption by doctors in Britain was similar to the national average in 1951, but the proportion had dropped dramatically to between one quarter to one half of the general population by 1971 [195]. The SMR for doctors from lung cancer was 35% of that expected for the general population [194].

Mental illness

It has been a commonly held belief that workers who are prone to psychiatric illness tend to have background of low socio-economic status and low educational achivement. Thus, they tend to work in low skill occupations [167,199]. This assumption has been challenged by Cooper [169] who suggests that the reaction to stress differs in white collar workers and blue collar workers in that the former reflects the pressure of work in mental illness whereas the latter do so in physical symptoms and illness.

Mental illness in doctors

Doctors are known to be hesitant in admitting their own illness. They may take it for granted that they are not supposed to be ill because they are physicians and they fail to realise that they are as susceptible to illness as their patients. The true prevalence of mental illness in doctors is much less known than for physical illness and the studies available appear to inflate the incidence. Most include those treated as ill as inpatients, representing more severe cases. In addition not only do doctors treat themselves but may also seek out a doctor colleague with particular expertise in that condition. This may distort the results described in the studies below.

In the past (1964 to 1972) there have been seven major series of published studies on doctors receiving treatment for mental illness, as summmarised in Table 4.1. The percentage diagnosed as having affective psychosis ranged from 21% to 40% and those with schizophrenia varied from 2% to 12%. Drug addiction and alcoholism were extremely common – in one series, 51% of the doctors under enquiry were found to be addicted to drugs or alcohol (see Table 4.1).

Table 4.1 Studies of mentally-ill doctors – diagnostic aspects

	Duffy & Litin [201] %	a'Brook et al. [202] %	Vincent et al. [203] %	Pond [204] %	Small et al. [205] %	Franklin [206] %	Jones [207] %
Affective psychosis	21	28	14	28	15	40	24
Alcoholism }		12	27	20	18	20	5
Drug dependence }	51 *	17	30	–	15	10	5
Neurosis	20	16	14	21	–	17	52
Schizophrenia	7	9	5	12	52 **	2	6
Personality disorder	7	13	4	–	–	4	3
Organic psychosis	9	5	5	7	–	8	1

* includes secondary diagnosis
** category of 'schizophrenic reactions'

Source [208]

Most of these studies are retrospective and show such a wide range of incidence that their accuracy must be questioned. One prospective study by Vaillant *et al.* [209] observed 47 medical student graduates, and matching controls, over a period of 30 years. During that period 17% were hospitalised for psychiatric illness, 34% underwent psychotherapy (control 19%), 36% used drugs, whilst only 22% of the control did so. Although the numbers here are small the trend is fairly consistent, and it agrees with other studies. A study on 89 male and 11 female doctor inpatients, showed that affective disorders and drug abuse were higher than in the general population [207]. The same study showed that the incidence of schizophrenia was slightly lower but manic depressive illness was twice as much in comparison with general hospital discharges. Neuroses and personality disorders were higher. Alcohol and drug addiction were three times that of the hospital population. It is also believed that GPs and psychiatrists have higher rates for the various problems mentioned above than do the rest of the medical profession [145].

In a well controlled epidemiological study, Murray [210] studied the admissions to, and discharges from all Scottish hospitals of male doctors aged 25 years and over. He compared them with the figures for all male non-doctor of social class 1. The overall mean annual first admission rate was 449 per 100,000 for male doctors and 205 per 100,000 for the non-medical males of social class 1. The rates were higher among doctors for all diagnostic categories except personality and behaviour disorders, but there was no significant difference between doctors and non-doctors for schizophrenia, other psychoses and neuroses. The study showed that the rates for drug dependence, alcoholism, and depression were significantly more common amongst doctors than non-doctors, particularly in middle age. Fifty-eight percent of all doctors hospitalised between the ages of 45 years and 54 years were found to be alcoholics.

The prevalence of mental illness in medical students is clearly shown in several studies. Bojar [211] reported that 25% of students seek psychiatric help before graduation from medical school. Pitts et al. [212] conducted structured psychiatric interviews to a random sample of 40 students at their medical school. It was found that 15% (6) received a psychiatric diagnosis including manic depressive cases, anxiety reaction and chronic alcoholism with histories ranging from 6 months to 12 years. Salmons [213] examined medical student records at a British university for the previous 25 years and discovered that 2.4% had been reported as developing a psychiatric disorder and 1% required hospitalization. She observed that total psychiatric morbidity was likely to be considerably higher since details of some of the students problems treated may not have been entered into the medical records.

Lloyd and Gartrell [214] estimated that between 15% and 25% of medical students met the criteria for a psychiatric diagnosis within their medical school. The difficulty with this study, as with many of the other such questionnaire surveys, is that response rates were low (39% of students replied), and only one medical school was investigated.

In a longitudinal study, Firth [215] used the 12 item version of the General Health Questionnaire (GHQ–12), a measure of perceived strain used in a number of occupational studies, at three British provincial universities for fourth year medical students. It was found that mean strain levels among medical students (11.66 on the GHQ–12) were higher than comparable groups within the normal population (8.67). Thirty percent of students fell into the psychiatric caseness category compared with 9.1% in a comparable sample of young employed men and women. This study makes its finding particularly important because of its high return rate (78.5%). Having said that it is worth noting the finding of an epidemiological survey by Vernon *et al.* [216], who found that non-respondents tended to be more depressed than respondents.

It may be possible that all these findings are demonstrations of high pressure levels in students as a whole rather than in medical students alone. Bjorksten *et al.* [217] compared medical students with other health-oriented student groups (dentists, pharmacists, nurses and allied professions) at their university. The finding was that medical students had a wide range of problems which were significantly more intense than the other groups.

It is possible that it is because medical students get less sleep, less time for recreation and work for longer hours that make them a vulnerable group. This is supported by a study by Friedman *et al.* [218] which showed that when interns were deprived of sleep they felt significantly more fatigue, more dejected, greater sadness and perceived themselves to develop several psycho-physiological abnormalities. The psychological problems reported were depression, difficulty in thinking, irritability, referentiality, depersonalization and recent memory deficit.

As well as the problem of sleep deprivation and other intrinsic stressors it is possible that the family history of medical students might contribute to their psychophysiological abnormalities. Valko and Clayton [219] studied 54 interns and found that 30% of them suffered from depression. Four of them had suicidal ideation, three had suicidal plan and six had marital difficulties with their depression. They found that the depressed interns had a positive family history of depression and a family history of suicidal attempts. Also Waring [220] claimed that for medical students the family history of mental illness, life experience and the personality before entering medical school are of greater importance in the formation of psychopathology than the occupational hazards of medical practice. Vaillant [109] found unstable childhood and adolescent adjustments as a critical factor in doctors with poor marriages, drug or alcohol abuse, or psychiatric difficulties.

Werner *et al.* [221] reported that interns whose personalities are well integrated and who have strong self-esteem may fare better than those with unresolved conflicts. Lief *et al.* [222] suggested that superior rated medical students cope better with their emotional difficulties and personality problems than the lower ranking students. Those lower ranking students tended to utilise neurotic defences in coping with stress arising from education and training. Nadleson and Notman [223] advise that "the factors affecting vulnerability, distress and symptom formation are complex: the nature, the number and magnitude of the stresses and individual personality factors and capacities must all be considered".

Doctors' job satisfaction

Studies on job satisfaction in different occupational groups revealed many factors are likely to contribute to poor job satisfaction. Kasl [167] established that low job satisfaction was related to non-participation in decision making, inability to provide feedback and lack of recognition of good performance. French and Caplan [90] considered that poor relationships with other members of the organisation could result in psychological strain in the form of lower job satisfaction.

Caplan *et al.* [168] attempted to identify the sources of stress among 23 different occupational groups. In summarising this work, Cooper [169] describes the differentiation of two separate groups of factors reported by white- and blue-collar workers as responsible for job dissatisfaction and ill health. For the professional and white-collar workers the major sources of stress were responsibility for people, job complexity and concentration, and high and variable workload. In white-collar workers the manifestations of stress were found more likely to be through mental ill health. For blue-collar workers, on the other hand, the set of stressors which are responsible for (ill) health related behaviours were: lack of job complexity, ambiguity about job future, role ambiguity and under-utilisation of abilities.

In the case of doctors, Mawardi [84] found that doctors were dissatisfied with their work because of heavy work load, not having personal free time and being on call. Clarke *et al.* [171], in their study of neonatologists found that the degrees of stress and job satisfaction were inversely correlated with each other. However, Linn *et al.* [68] found that doctors expressed their work satisfaction with the diversity of patients seen, as well as with their ability to derive personal gratification from patient care. Rankin and colleagues have suggested that GPs derive pleasure from the exercise of their technical skills [74] but the social and the administrative aspect of their job may lead to dissatisfaction.

Cartwright's studies [9,73] on GPs have provided some information on those aspects of practice work that GPs found frustrating. In 1977 more doctors said that they enjoyed the diversity of their work and more expressed appreciation of their freedom and independence. The proportion of respondents who specifically mentioned that they enjoyed 'being their own master' and having 'freedom and independence' changed from 10% to 26%. There was an increase in the proportion who said they felt frustrated because they did not have enough time to do their own work properly.

Cartwright and Anderson [9] view that although there was no change in surgery consultation rates and there was a drop in home visits the majority of doctors felt they were more busy in 1977 than they had been ten years previously. They suggest that the increase in secretaries, nurses and other attached staff working with GPs may have enabled them to delegate some tasks, but coordinating the efforts of a team takes time and energy. In both the studies of Cartwright only about 10% said that they were not enjoying their work. Forty percent of the GPs in 1977 felt frustrated by trivial and inappropriate consultations compared with 48% in 1964. In both the 1964 and 1977 studies about a quarter of GPs felt that 50% or more surgery consultations were trivial or unnecessary. This finding suggests that there has been little change in orientation between 1964 and 1977.

Melville [172] has studied the job satisfaction of GPs and quality of prescribing. She views that low job satisfaction is associated with higher levels of prescribing of certain drugs with potential adverse side effects. She suggests that job dissatisfaction appears to be correlated with frustration and she gave two reasons for this. According to her the personality characteristics of some GPs might not match to the requirement of the GP work; and secondly, certain aspects of the GP's task could lead to dissatisfaction. From our pilot study [60] of 101 GPs in the North West of England it was found that the GP's job is the source of considerable job satisfaction. Freedom to determine working methods and the amount of responsibility in the job showed the highest levels, whilst recognition for good work, and hours of work are the aspects of the job that gives least satisfaction. Also from the same study it was found that GPs were dissatisfied about their poor pay. It would appear that most GPs feel they lack recognition and praise, whether from their colleagues or patients. GPs felt significantly more dissatisfied with the job in 1990 than they were before the introduction of the new contract [64]. McCranie *et al.* [173], in a national survey of family physicians, found that time pressures and financial costs of operating a practice were the major sources of job dissatisfaction.

One of the components of job satisfaction is prestige. In Cartwright's study when GPs were asked about their prestige within the medical profession, they thought it had gone up. This may be due to the influence of the Royal College of General

Practitioners and the emphasis on training giving GPs more confidence, which in turn led to more satisfaction. In a study Mechanic [174] found that almost half of British GPs were either 'not very satisfied' or 'quite dissatisfied' with general practice, and 24% expressed that half or more of patient consultations were trivial, unnecessary or inappropriate. In contrast only a small proportion of American practitioners (4%) declared feelings of dissatisfaction, and only 9–13% felt that half or more consultations were trivial or inappropriate. Mechanic describes the characteristics and orientations of British GPs which confirms the impression that British GPs with high social orientation are likely to be more satisfied than those GPs with low social orientation, and less likely to consider consultations as trivial or inappropriate.

Suicide in doctors

A doctor's suicide is a devastating waste of human resources. Yet British government statistics show explicitly high suicide rates for doctors as compared with other professionals such as lawyers, school teachers, the clergy and, of course, the general public [145]. The 1970–1972 Decennial Supplement [194] revealed that three major diseases from which doctors are more likely to die than the general population are suicide (SMR–335), cirrhosis (SMR–311), and accidents (SMR–180). In Britain, doctors are nearly 3.5 times more likely to commit suicide than in general population [224].

An American study reviewed all the Obituary notices in the Journal of the American Medical Association between 1965 and 1967 [225]. Two hundred and forty nine suicides were reported giving an annual suicide risk for doctors of 33 per 100,000, close to the average for all white males in the USA. Steppacher and Mausner [226] studied 530 deaths (489 male and 41 female physicians) by suicide in a 5½-year period (March 1965 to August 1970). They noted that the suicide rate for male physicians was 1.15 times than that of the total male population and for female physicians it was three times.

Rose and Roscow [227] reviewed all death certificates of males in California from 1959 to 1961 and revealed that physicians, and health care workers as a group, are twice as suicide prone as the general population. The doctors who tend to kill themselves were relatively young (half the suicides in male doctors studied by Rose and Roscow occurred between 35 and 54 years of age).

The chairman of the American Psychiatric Association's impaired physician committee has suggested that female physicians in particular tend to be more vulnerable to suicide than male physicians. As noted earlier Steppacher and Mausner's study [226] reported a suicide rate for female physicians three times that expected on the basis of population statistics. In their study more female physicians' suicide occurred during the training period than male physicians and more of the female physicians were single. Craig and Pitts [228] found a fourfold excess of suicide among women doctors compared with the general population.

In a study of graduates and non-graduates of a medical school from 1948 to 1964, Thomas [229] found that 3.7% of 1337 subjects died prematurely; 3.1% were graduates and 11.2% non-graduates. Suicide was the most frequent cause (17 cases). Sakinofsky [117] looked at data (Office of Population Censuses and Surveys, England and Wales) on the marital state of the 55 male doctors (age 25–64) who committed suicide during 1970–1972. He discovered that unmarried and divorced doctors tend to be more suicidal (age group 35–54). Twice as many doctors among the suicides remained unmarried than among other living doctors. However, the small sample size makes it unwise to conclude too much from this data. But we may speculate that there is some form of threat.

In 1986 the American Psychiatric Association and the American Medical Association co-sponsored a study to determine suicidal death in physicians. A comparison was made between physicians who committed suicide with a control group who died from natural causes. It was found that 219 physicians were reported to have killed themselves between 1982 and 1984. Of the original 219, 142 interviews were obtained from relatives. The family members of control groups were interviewed: family members of those dying from natural causes (68) and those dying of ambiguous circumstances (33). Of the 142 suicidal cases, 129 were male and 13 were female. Sixty-nine percent of the entire group was married or living as married at the time of suicide whereas only five of the female physicians were married. Sargent [230] interpreted that the results "implicated biological heredity and premorbid personality as causative factors of suicide. The stresses particular to life in medicine are seen as aggravating factors which may differently affect women". This study showed that presuicidal physicians show some mental health problems including prior suicidal threats, chronic illness at the time of death, a history of psychiatric treatment, self-prescribing drugs, prior suicide attempts, prior psychiatric hospitalization, violence to spouse, sexual problems in marriage, acknowledged drug abuse, smoking, blaming self for illness and financial loss in the two years before death [231].

Another possibile reason for suicide amongst physicians may be due to the wrong choice of career. Schwartz *et al.* [232] found that students who were inclined towards artistic and literary careers before entering medicine were more vulnerable to the signs and symptoms of strain and expressed significantly more suicidal ideation than those students who were inclined to pursue a scientific career.

It is clear from the above evidence that doctors are exceedingly prone to suicide. Clearly, the recording of suicide is minimal [227], for it is uncertain how many suicides go unrecognised or are reported as accidental deaths. A bigger longitudinal study based on psychological testing of present medical students may provide more detail on the specific traits of those who later commit suicide.

Drug abuse in doctors

It has been emphasized by many investigators that drug abuse is an occupational hazard for doctors. Norwood East [233] reported that of the 383 known addicts in the UK at that time, 21.4% were doctors. The General Medical Council (GMC) reported that between September 1980 and August 1981, out of 51 doctors investigated, 19 were classified as drug addicts or alcoholics [234]. The medical profession in the UK has expressed its serious concern about drug dependency and alcoholism amongst doctors [235,236].

In the USA, one study reported a 20-year follow-up of 45 physicians who were originally described as 'psychologically unsound'. On follow-up, it was found that a large number of them continuously engaged in self-medicating with drugs or regularly abusing alcohol (1.6 times more frequent among doctors than for a comparable group of non-doctors) [209,237]. The reasons given by addicted physicians were overwork, fatigue and physical illness. It was found that doctors inclined to prescribe for themselves which often leads to concommitant drug addiction [210,238]. Usually such physicians are reluctant to be treated and sometimes commit suicide [210].

In addition to the series of mentally ill doctors previously reviewed, in all of which drug addiction was common (see Table 4.1), drug addiction was claimed to be present in 17% of doctors [202]. According to the US Commissioner of Narcotics [240] the drug addiction rate in the general population was 1:3000. A professor of psychiatry at the University of Arizona (reported in Medical World News, 1984) viewed that more than 4000 physicians in the USA were known addicts.

There have also been older studies of drug-dependent doctors [241–243]. Putnam and Ellingwood [244] followed up 68 addicted doctors discharged from Lexington Hospital and found that the major drugs of addiction were morphine, mepiridine and barbiturates. Green *et al.* [245] in a study of 46 Virginia physicians covering the period 1947–1974 found that the main drugs used in order of frequency were 'hard' narcotics, ataraxics and stimulants, used alone or in combination with narcotics. The most frequently addicted were family practitioners and internists.

It would appear that there is some evidence of drug abuse related to the stresses of doctors' occupations. However, Green *et al.* [245] viewed that a combination of predisposing personality disorder and the easy availability of drugs were the main reasons of drug abuse among physicians.

Alcoholism

Drinking alcohol is a recognised serious reaction to psychosocial and occupational stress. Margolis *et al.* [102], in a study in the USA, interviewed over 1500 workers in a variety of occupations, and discovered a positive relationship between escapist drinking and a number of specific job stressors. Those experiencing high job stress drank more than those in occupations where there was less job stress. Hurrel and Kroes [246] considered that the presence of high levels of stress at work can facilitate some individuals to resort to heavy drinking as a coping technique.

Alcoholism in general is on the increase, with admissions to alcoholism units in British hospitals increasing from under 6000 in 1966 to over 8000 in 1974 [169]. Deaths from alcoholism have trebled between 1965 to 1980, and admission to psychiatric units for alcoholism treatment has doubled for men and trebled for women in recent years [247,248]. Deaths from cirrhosis of the liver have increased since 1961, especially in Scotland (see Figure 4.1).

Alcoholism in doctors

Britain is experiencing an upsurge of alcohol dependency and doctors would seem to be more susceptible to it. A study by Murray [249] in Scotland showed that the first admission rate for alcohol dependence was 2.7 times higher among doctors than among controls (social class 1).

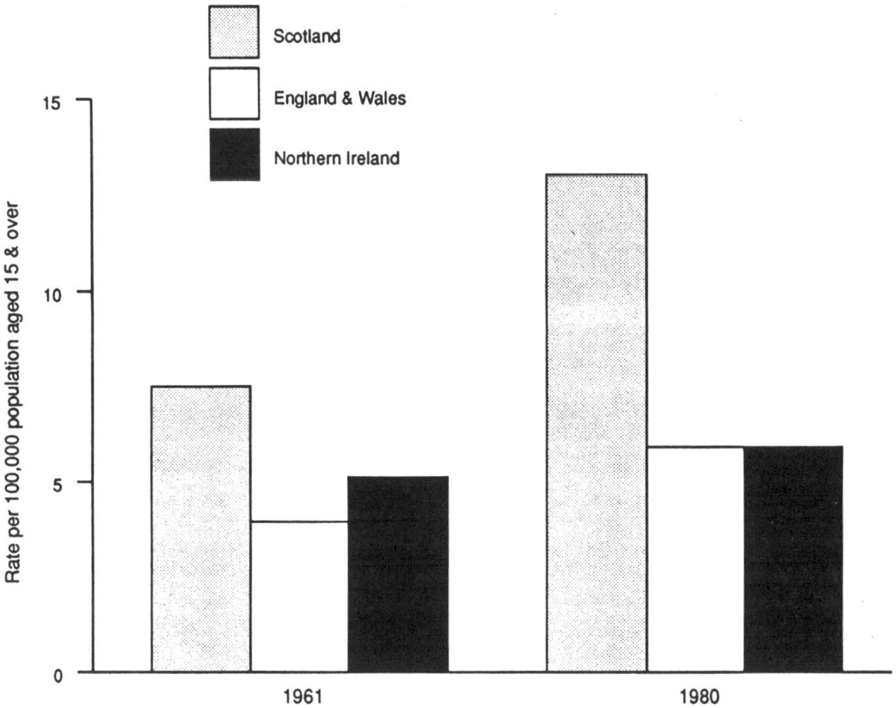

Figure 4.1. Deaths from cirrhosis of the liver in men in Scotland, England and Wales, and Northern Ireland (Social Trends, 1983, Chart 7.9). Source: [14]

The medical professional is especially susceptible to cirrhosis, suicide, poisonings, accidents, and alcohol addiction [66,145,208,250]. The death rates of doctors from liver cirrhosis is 3.1 time greater than that of the general population of England and Wales. In terms of absolute numbers of affected doctors alcoholism is much more important than drug dependence in Britain.

In the USA the estimate that 6–10% of the drinking American population became alcoholics [245] would be undoubtedly true for physicians, the upper rate being more likely [209,251]. It was found that 13,000–22,000 doctors in the USA were alcohol dependent at some stage in their career [238]. Bissel and Jones [238] interviewed 98 American doctors who were members of the Alcoholic Anonymous (AA) and had refrained for a minimum of one year. These 98 physicians had accumulated a total of

219 arrests and 170 jailings. From this and Murray's [208] study it was also shown that only a few alcoholic doctors have a family history of alcoholism or psychiatric disorders.

Literature on impaired physicians in the USA showed that in 1980, 1608 impaired physicians were in contact with the State Medical Society Programmes. Drug and alcohol abuse problems appear more common in male doctors [252]. Gomberg [253], on a national level in the USA reported that there were approximately 4 to 5 male alcoholics for every female alcoholic. In the UK, Allibone and his colleagues [66] estimated that there may be as many as 3000 practising GPs who are alcoholics, while many others may show other signs of stress.

Smoking

Not only is smoking related to the incidence of CHD but it is also associated with neuroticism and anxiety [254]. Doctors were one of the first groups to give up smoking once its harmful effects were known [194]. According to Lazarus [55] smoking can be seen as a form of palliative coping which provides temporary relief. Hence, giving up smoking may promote health but residual tension may remain which in turn influence the behaviours in a damaging way such as excessive alcohol drinking and self-prescribing of drugs [145,208,250,256]. Lee [257] also explained that cigarette smoking may have helped doctors to cope with stress temporarily.

Divorce

Over the past 30 years the divorce rate has risen steeply, with at least one in four marriages in Britain and one in three in America ending in divorce within 15 years, but with three-quarters of divorcees marrying again within three years [258]. Although it is acknowledged that divorce rates are on the increase in general, several researchers maintain that divorce in doctors is not more common than the rest of the population [111,112]. On the other hand marriages and sexual relationships in doctors are often unsatisfactory [84,109].

Nadelson and Nutman [129] cited Roscow and Rose's [259] study of doctors' divorces. The divorce rate in female doctors was higher than male doctors and higher than for the general population, whereas the divorce rate in male doctors was lower than for most male professionals and men in general. The ratio of divorces for female doctors compared with male doctors was 3 to 2. This may be due to the pressures of the family and the job and other dual career issues in the female doctors.

Divorced doctors are more likely to commit suicide than those who are widowed or single and least likely among married doctors. While in the general population divorcees are three times as suicide prone as the married, divorced doctors are 13 times more likely to kill themselves than their married colleagues, though other individuals in the same social class also show this greatly increased suicide risk with marital breakdown [256]

Conclusion

From studies on physical and mental health it seems that physicians are far better than the general population in withstanding physical illness but are less resistant to psychiatric illness, alcoholism, drug addiction and suicide. This suggests that their defences or ways of coping operate satisfactorily in conditions leading to physical illness but not so in psychiatric illness. Perhaps familiarity with death lessens the fear of dying, and the easy availability of drugs makes the physician more prone to addiction and suicide.

This evidence suggests, therefore, that GPs, as members of the medical profession, may be subject to occupational stress.

Although much has been written about the possible causes (e.g. heavy workload, dealing with the terminally ill, excessive paperwork, etc.) of this stress, little large scale empirical work is available to substantiate, or otherwise, these claims. The authors decided that this was an area which required further investigation in order that the GPs problems, pressures and stress outcomes could be recognised and tackled. The following three chapters describe our studies and their results.

Chapter 5 – THE INTERVIEWS WITH DOCTORS

It was felt to be essential to adopt both a qualitative and a quantitative approach to data collection in this study. The qualitative approach was in the form of in-depth interviews. The quantitative approach consisted of a survey questionnaire based on the analysis of these interviews.

The ultimate aim of the research was to identify sources of occupational and psycho-social stress among GPs, that is, to determine which, if any, aspects of the way of life give rise to subjectively experienced feelings of stress.

This chapter is devoted to the comments made by GPs during our interviews and the next chapter covers the main, quantitative survey.

In-depth interviews were carried out on a random sample of 42 GPs at the end of 1987 in different parts of England with the aim of investigating the major sources of stress and levels of stress experienced by GPs. Each interview lasted from 30 to 60 minutes, and covered the following areas:

- Potential causes of stress at work
- Potential causes of stress at home in relation to work
- Drinking and smoking habits of the GPs

Out of 42 GPs, 28 were male and 14 female, 30 were principals and 12 were trainees. The age range varied between 28 and 60. There were 15 overseas and 27 UK qualified GPs. Out of 42, 34 were married, four were single, one divorced, one widowed and two living together. Seven GPs were in solo practices and 35 were in group practices. There were 28 urban practice GPs, six rural practice GPs, and eight mixed practice GPs (see Appendix 2). The interview format was unstructured at the beginning but, as a result of the responses of the interviewees, became more structured.

Interview analysis

When the GPs were asked to what extent they found their job stressful, all of them indicated that they experienced moderate to high stress at work. The method of descriptive statistics was adopted in order to give percentage estimates of responses to items in the sample population. Table 5.1 shows that time pressure, emergency calls during surgery hours, night calls, telephone calls during the night and early morning and dealing with problem patients were isolated as the leading causes of stress.

Comments made by the GPs during the interviews suggested that interruptions of any kind and time pressure were considered as very stressful. Examples of such comments, out of which the stressors have been extracted, are now given.

"I do not really have that much of a problem in doing the surgeries. The problem starts when interruptions of telephone calls, partners' interruptions and staff interruptions encroach upon me. Another irritating matter is to see extra patients. We have an appointment system but some patients just walk in at any moment without an appointment expecting to be seen by a doctor. In addition, the appointment is usually for five minutes but some patients take 20 to 30 minutes just to talk about their non-medical problems. Then I am pushed for time and fall behind the surgery appointments for the rest of the patients and other commitments after the surgery. This is very stressful."

"Often the telephone calls come seconds after entering through the front door. At other times it is annoying to return home from one visit, only to receive a request from their next door neighbour."

"I find it most irritating and frustrating to wake up from a deep sleep during the night and early morning to answer the telephone when patients may be ringing for trivial reasons. I just don't know how I cope with it. It is tiring, it is exhausting, it is irritating, it is fatiguing."

"When I was working in the hospital I was able to transfer the responsibility to my senior colleagues and after 5 pm I did not have to take any responsibility at all unless I was on call. But here I am responsible for my patients lives 24 hours a day, even after the evening surgery. I am unable to relax completely at home because there is a possibility that the telephone might ring. I may be watching television but my sixth sense remains alert to receive telephone calls."

"I feel that most of the night calls for visits are for minor ailments which, with a bit of common sense, could be managed by the patients themselves or their relatives. They have no patience to wait until the next day's surgery. Some patients have the habit of asking for a visit soon after the end of the evening surgery, knowing very well that they could have been seen during the surgery hours and obtain the medicine while the chemists were open. I have seen this myself that after seeing a patient during early evening hours the prescription still lies on the fireplace or the windowsill until the next afternoon. This shows how the patients use us. I don't mind doing night visits for genuine illness but unnecessary calls during unsocial hours drive me mad."

"It is very annoying when calls come for emergency visits half-way through the surgery. No matter how well you organise the surgery, there remains the uncertainty of this kind. I feel guilty to leave the patients in the waiting room, but at the same time I am obliged to attend the emergency calls."

Table 5.1 Interview sample: stressful situations

To what extent do you find your job stressful and what elements of your job cause unhappiness in your family life?	Percentage of total sample ($n = 42$)
1. Time pressure	95
2. Emergency calls during surgery hours	95
3. Night calls	93
4. Dealing with problem patients	93
5. Coping with phone calls during night and early morning	88
6. Interruption of family life by telephone	88
7. 24 hours responsibility for patients' lives	88
8. Demands of the job on family life	85
9. Practice administration	85
10. Unrealistically high expectations by others of your role	85
11. Arranging admissions	81
12. Remaining alert when on call	81
13. Demands of the job on social life	76
14. Dividing time between spouse and patients	74
15. Partner on holiday	74
16. Hospital referrals and paperwork	71
17. Home visits	64
18. Conducting surgery	64
19. Coping with numerous journals and newsletters	59
20. Worrying about patients' complaints	57
21. Increased demands by patients and relatives for second opinions from hospital specialists	52
22. Dealing with terminally ill and their relatives	45
23. Dealing with relatives as patients	40
24. Dealing with friends as patients	40
25. No appreciation of your work by patients	40
26. Finding a locum	33
27. Adverse publicity in the press	30
28. Visiting in extremely adverse weather conditions	28
29. Coping with new technology	26
30. Fear of assault during night visits	23
31. Conflict with partners in a group practice	23
32. Examining patients of opposite sex	4
33. Daily contact with dying and chronically ill patients	4
34. Working environment	4
35. Taking work home (paperwork, etc.)	2
36. Taking several samples in a short time	2
37. Lack of emotional support at home especially from spouse	2
38. Driving in relation to your work	2

> "My wife complains that I come home 'emotionally drained' and I have no time to spend with her. One way she is right because sometimes soon after entering the home I get on the telephone to answer the bleep which went off on my way home. Discussing the patients' problems on the phone does not amuse my wife and children. While she has been waiting to have dinner with me, I may have to go back again to do the call even though I am hungry. Many times telephone calls interrupt my dinner, sleep, family and social life."

> "With heavy workload and time pressure I hardly get any time to open the medical journals and newsletters. There is so much advancement in modern medicine, that unless I keep up with the journals I may miss important issues. I try to go through them during nights and weekends but at the cost of my family life."

The following quote, however, suggests that time pressure for a GP is unavoidable. A GP cited:

> "There is always shortage of time for me. There is too little personal time, continuous on call responsibilities and demands of the work load and too many things to do . . . I do not like the occasions when psychiatric patients resist admissions. This requires compulsory admission under a section. This is extremely time consuming as liaison between social worker and psychiatric consultant must have to be established. The patient has to be seen before the section papers can be signed by the GP, social worker and the consultant. This means additional work load which is unpredictable and interrupts the time table . . . I always try to be organised but in situations like this everything gets messed up."

Likewise comments made on problem patients:

> "I find very often that some patients come to see me without any medical problem but just to talk to someone. Some others come to obtain a letter of recommendation for rehousing, obtaining additional benefits from social security departments on grounds for which they are not entitled to. I feel my medical education was not meant to solve these non-medical problems."

> "It is ridiculous that the patients expect me to do many things that I am not supposed to do at all. I have to do unnecessary calls, on top of that I have to collect the medicine for them from the chemist."

> "The most harrassing situation in General Practice is dealing with problem patients, invariably patients with psychiatric disorders and those frequent attenders who do not suffer from real illness. There are some patients who instead of attending the surgery would ring outside the surgery hours presenting their problems as an emergency on every occasion."

"The majority of stress, I find comes from difficult and angry patients who do not understand our role or the limitations to medical health, particularly regarding out of hours work, and immediate treatment, and hospital admission. Patients seem to think they know what they should be getting even when they have no idea. One is tempted to give in, for the sake of peace and quiet."

"The problem patients attend the surgery more frequently, often with vague and trivial complaints and consume at least 20 to 30 minutes of my time unnecessarily. I am not here to wipe their tears."

"The patients expectations have risen to such an extent that they want us to solve their physical, psychological, social and even their financial problems. What help can I offer if someone comes to me and says her husband has been away with another lady? There are many problems which can be solved by non-medical personnel instead of our time being wasted."

"Many a times patients who do not have their own transport expect us to visit them at home even though they are quite capable of attending the surgery by using public transport. These types of unnecessary and ingenuine calls annoy me but it is difficult to refuse as the patient could put a complaint which would create unnecessary hassle."

Non-medical problems are welcomed by some GPs as a variety in general practice but others feel that it should not be their responsibility.

"I find patients coming to see me more often to obtain letters for housing, social benefits, for schools, cancellation of holiday, etc. They expect me to support their social needs and sometimes to transfer their inconvenience to a medical illness so that they can cancel their holiday and get their money back from the insurance company."

"To me the problem patients are a nuisance. They just waste my time which I could utilise for genuine needs. The NHS set-up is stopping people being self-reliant and this prevents the more needy getting the help they need."

More comments made by some GPs on administrative responsibility:

"I never had any training on practice administration during my medical education and never expected to do this sort of paperwork. I find that I am being forced to do this, which I don't really enjoy."

"You may think that one just sees patients and hands out prescriptions. There is a great deal of paperwork to be done for admission to hospital, and referrals to out-patients department and many other forms to complete. We have to claim for every item of service we provide, by filling in different forms, otherwise we lose out financially."

Junior partners may find it difficult to motivate senior partners with their innovative ideas. As one GP says:

> "We thought that by installing a computer system our workload will be dramatically reduced, but instead it takes a tremendous amount of time to handle it. Now I find that my senior partners do not take any interest in the computer system. The responsibility for its maintenance is imposed on me as I am the most junior. Indirectly I am being blamed for taking the initiative in its installation and the amount of capital investment involved. These additional administrative workloads take up all my time which I expected to be shared with others, so that I could give more time for my patients."

To satisfy all the staff in an organisation is not an easy job as much depends on individual staff's attitude and behaviour.

> "Many of my patients have complained to me about the impolite manner of one of my secretaries at the reception desk. Another secretary whose husband is a union leader, talks of nothing but labour laws, including holiday entitlement, sick leave, pay rises, etc. These matters put me off."

Comments made by some GPs suggested that during their partner(s) holiday the remaining partners on duty were under stress.

> "During the summer holiday when everybody wants to take time off, it creates chaos in the surgery organisation. It is not easy to find a reliable locum who would satisfy our patients the way we try to. In one instance, there were two partners on holiday and the third one was suddenly taken ill. The practice manager had not managed to fix a locum. I was the only one doing four people's work. On that evening I finished the surgery at 8.30 pm and still had some visits to do. I don't know how I coped but I felt that I was on the verge of cracking up."

> "We have an agreement in our partnership to cover each other during holidays. It is not too bad when only one partner is on holiday but at times when more than one is away I feel the pressure. Even when we employ a locum, some patients, especially females, create problems as they only want to be seen by their own doctor and are less willing to consult partners or locums."

Further comments made by some GPs on dealing with terminally ill patients and their relatives, and increased demands by patients and relatives for second opinions from hospital specialists:

> "I find it hard work to care for the dying patients and chronically ill. Their relatives are more demanding even after knowing full well that there is no possibility of a cure and death is inevitable. The patient himself has unrealistically high expectations from me that I should be able to create a miracle to cure his disease or send him to a specialist to do the same."

"Often some caring relatives show their willingness to care for the terminally ill patients but once they feel that it is a bit too much for them, there is an immediate demand on us to arrange admission to a hospital or a hospice without any delay."

Many doctors expressed their unhappiness for not being appreciated for their work by their patients. For example, one GP commented:

"Sometimes I get called out to do night calls at unsocial hours and in adverse weather conditions which could have waited until the next day. There have been several assaults on GPs during night visits which scares me but I am forced to do these calls. After all the trouble we take, we do not get appreciation of our work by patients."

Some comments on remaining alert while on call, and taking several samples in a short time:

"In the hospital there are technicians to collect blood samples and to do ECG but here I have to do all this myself within a limited period. Besides this I have to take other samples, for example, cervical smears, etc., within a short period during surgery."

"The uncertainty about the content of 'on call' days makes me really unhappy. Any moment the telephone might ring. Even though there are less than three calls in an 'on call' day, I have to wait until eleven at night."

Similarily for examining patients of the opposite sex and worrying about patients' complaints, the following comments were made:

"While examining the private parts of female patients I always try to ask my secretary to be a chaperone. But there are occasions when she is busy at her desk and I have to get on with the job. In these circumstances I do not feel comfortable in examining such patients. I have always this fear that a young woman patient may make allegations against me for malpractice, even if I do not do anything wrong because of her dissatisfaction with events unrelated to this."

"The younger the woman patient the more I feel awkward to examine her. When I used to examine patients of the opposite sex in hospital, a chaperone was readily available but here sometimes I have to examine a patient without a chaperone, which I don't like."

Some GPs commented on the demands made by the job on their family and social life:

"Sometimes I bring paperwork home, which drives my wife mad . . . She says 'why don't you have a bed in the surgery and one for your secretary so that she can answer your telephone calls, instead of asking me to do it'."

"My wife expects me to spend more time with her. I wish I could give a bit more time to her and my children. But the profession I have chosen is so demanding that I can't afford to cut short my duty towards my patients."

Commitment to work and to family should be balanced. Excess involvement in one is likely to cause neglect to the other.

"My wife and children always complain that I promise them to come home immediately after evening surgery to have dinner together but I have not been able to do it for the last ten years. By the time I finish evening surgery and come home, my children are almost ready to go to bed. I am unable to spend time with them."

"I find it a cause of frustration that the night of our wedding anniversary had to coincide with my duty night for the practice this year because of my senior partner's sudden illness. I don't blame my wife for being furious but I was helpless."

"Some patients wake up during the night with a physical problem but are sympathetic to me by not disturbing me at that hour. I would have been happy to attend such patients at that time rather than being called out in the early morning when I have to get myself ready and prepare the children to be dropped at the child minder."

"I conduct my own patients' deliveries in the GP unit at the local hospital. This means being called out to the maternity unit at any hour of the day including in the middle of surgery, from bed and even from the local pub, while I am with my friends."

Comments made by GPs on conflict with partners:

"I am the most junior partner in my practice. I feel that I am being forced to do the work that I don't believe in. I have been passed on a large list of patients for regular monthly visits. I simply think that this system is a waste of time. Recently it has been imposed on me to conduct a diabetic clinic without even my consent."

"I joined a group practice after my training but could manage only to stay there for three months. Two senior partners were hardly doing any surgery work and virtually did not do any home visits. I think they enjoyed too much their pipes and golf. It was impossible to motivate them with new ideas. Additional surgery, home visits and more weekends on-call were imposed on me. I could not cope with newsletters, journals or any research work. In the end I had to leave. Now I have full satisfaction as a single-handed GP."

Comments on adverse publicity in the press and unrealistically high expectations by others of their role:

> "One of the things I am most scared of is publicity in the press without any basis. Dissatisfied patients can blow up things in the paper as a revenge. These things happen more in the city areas."

> "Just before the evening surgery I developed a sore throat and fever. One of the senior partners in the practice noticed my infirmity but advised that I should take two paracetamol tablets and conduct the surgery as he had done the same thing in the past."

What do GPs dislike about their job?

When asked 'What do you dislike about your job', the most items listed by GPs were 'emergency calls during surgery hours', 'night calls', 'interruption of family life by telephone', 'practice administration', 'hospital referrals and paper work' (see Table 5.2).

Table 5.2 The interview sample: job dislikes

What do you dislike about your job	Percentage of total sample ($n=42$)
Emergency calls during surgery hours	97
Night calls	95
Interruption of family life by telephone	92
Practice administration	90
Hospital referrals and paperwork	90
Dealing with relatives and friends as patients	71
Dealing with problem patients	47

What change would GPs like to see?

On the issue of 'how to improve general practice', 47% of the interview sample suggested that there should be an introduction of administrative training courses for GPs (see Table 5.3), and even better, that this should be available during training in medical schools. Forty-five percent of the interview sample suggested that there should be improved financial reward for out-of-hour work. In addition 42% of the GPs interviewed said 'social orientation' during medical training would help them to solve many of the problems of the patients rather than purely technical skills training.

Table 5.3 The interview sample: how to improve general practice

What can be done to improve general practice	Percentage of total sample ($n=42$)
Training in practice administration	47
Improved financial reward for out-of-hours calls	45
Training in 'social orientation' rather than technical	42
Improve public education – not to waste doctor's time	28
More resources should be available to GPs. NHS cuts indirectly affecting GPs	28
Less interference from government and FHSAs	11

Table 5.4 Interview sample: smoking habit

Number of cigarettes a day	Percentage of total sample ($n=42$)
None	97
1 – 10 a day	2
11 – 20 a day	4
21 – 30 a day	0
31 – 40 a day	0

Do GPs drink and smoke?

In order to discover the smoking habit of the GPs, the interview sample were asked: 'Do you smoke? If so, how many a day?' Only 4% of the interview sample said they smoked an average of 20 cigarettes a day (see Table 5.4). Table 5.5 shows that an occasional drink was most common for GPs (97%). Twenty-three percent of the interview sample said that they had 1–2 drinks a day regularly. Of these who drank 1–2 drinks regularly, 81% claimed they did so because of work stress and the rest for personal reasons or habits. However because some did not like to talk about their drinking habits the reliability of this data is questionable.

Table 5.5 Interview sample: drinking habit

Number of drinks	Percentage of total sample ($n=42$)
Teetotal	2
An occasional drink	97
Several drinks a week	95
Regularly 1 or 2 drinks a day	23
Regularly 3 to 6 drinks a day	0
Regularly more than 6 drinks a day	0

In summary, the analysis of the qualitative data provided a rich source of stressors in GPs which proved invaluable in terms of the formulation of the survey questionnaire used in the study described next.

Chapter 6 – THE STUDY AND ITS FINDINGS

In this chapter we describe the full-scale study and its findings. This study aimed to determine how satisfied GPs are with their jobs, which aspects of the job GPs report as causing stress and their mental well-being. A pilot study was carried out first where a total of 200 questionnaires were distributed to GPs from a random sample of 72 practices in the Greater Manchester area. One hundred and eight questionnaires were returned, of which 101 could be analysed (a response rate of 50.5%). Of the sample 42 were group practices and 30 single-handed GPs. Men accounted for 81.2% of the sample, a figure close to the National sample average in 1980 (83%) and other available data [14]. The results of the pilot study have been published elsewhere [63]. For the main study a package of questionnaires (see Appendix 1) was sent to a random sample of 4000 GPs throughout the country. They were distributed by 20 Family Practitioner Committees (FPCs) during November 1987, selected to reflect a representative sample of practices in terms of urban, rural, social mix area and other demographic characteristics. Of the 4000 sent out 1928 were returned (a response rate of 48.2%) of which 1817 were complete enough for statistical analysis. Those excluded had either substantially incomplete sections or arrived after the cut-off date for analysis. The response rate was above average as compared with similar occupational stress studies [260]. Anonymity was considered essential to protect the identify of the doctors and to ensure the completeness of the responses.

Personal and job demographics

Gender

A total of 1469 (80.9%) males and 343 (18.9%) females returned the questionnaire. Although it is not possible to make exact comparisons with national figures these seem to reflect the balance with the profession. In 1970 only 10% of GPs were female, 90% were male. But in 1980, there were 83% male and 17% female GPs in England (see Appendix 3).

Age

The peak age of the respondents was in the range of 35–44 and then declined. The majority of respondents fell into the younger age group (25–44 years category). The age distribution of the GPs in this study is also roughly close to the national sample except for the over 60 and over 70 groups (see Appendix 4).

Figure 6.1 shows the age and sex composition of doctors in the research sample. Women were concentrated in the younger age groups. Wilkin *et al.* [261] in their Manchester sample of GPs, also found that 67% of women were below 40 years of age compared with 42% of men.

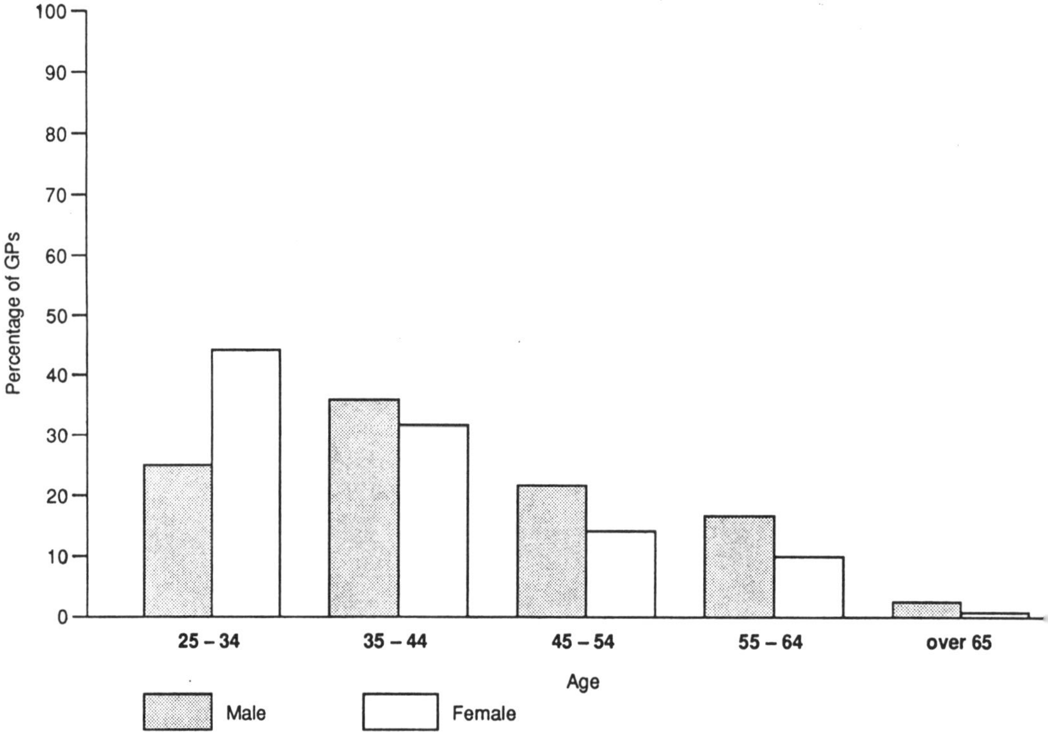

Figure 6.1. The age and sex distribution of the sample

Marital status

It was found that 87.4% (1588) of the respondents were married or lived with a partner and 11.9% (217) were single, divorced, separated, widowed or re-married (see Appendix 5). Thus the majority of GPs remained married and although divorce rates are on the increase in the general population [258], divorce in doctors is not more common than in the general population [111]. Higher percentages of women were single, widowed, divorced and cohabiting. The divorce rate for female doctors is higher than for male doctors (see Chapter 4) and this supports our finding.

Place of qualification and post-graduate qualification

It was found that 88.4% of GPs were qualified in the UK and 11.2% had received their first degrees overseas. The 1970 figures are very close to our samples but not 1980 figures (see Appendix 6). The percentage of female GPs who qualified in the UK was far greater than the percentage of female GPs who qualified overseas.

The majority of the respondents (70.8%) have obtained post-graduate qualifications (see Appendix 7). There was little difference in the percentage of male and female GPs with post-graduate qualifications.

Job

It was found that the percentage of principal GPs (96.5%) was much higher than the trainee GPs (3.5%) (see Appendix 8). The percentage of trainees was higher among female GPs. This may suggest that more female doctors are now choosing general practice as their preferred career.

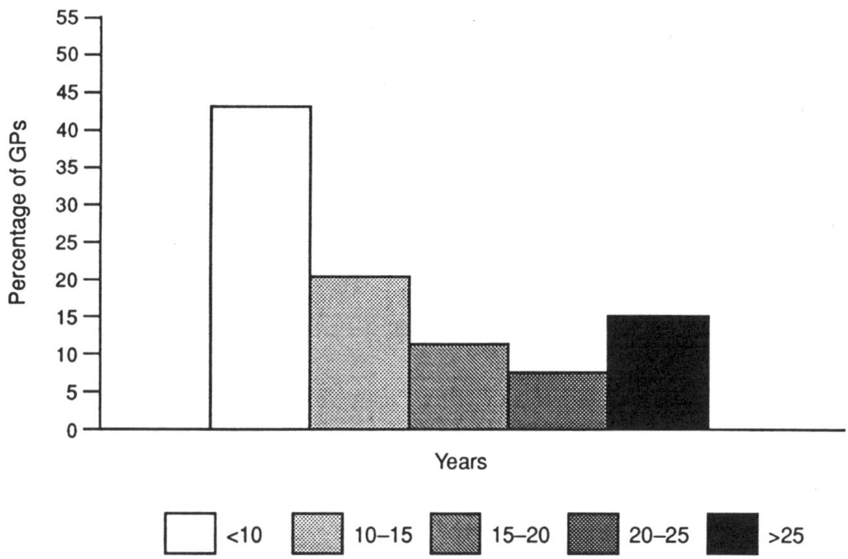

Figure 6.2. Years in general practice for the whole group

Practice type

As noted in Chapter 1 the tendency towards group practices has been increasing over the last two to three decades and most of the GPs in this sample were from group practices (see Appendix 9).

Experience in general practice

Interestingly a large number of the respondents (63.6%) had less than 10 and up to 15 years experience in general practice (see Figure 6.2). Thus the sample contains more younger GPs with less experience (see Appendix 10). There is a marked contrast between male and female GPs in their experience in general practice. Only 38.5% of the sample of male GPs had spent less than 10 years in general practice compared with 64.1% of their female colleagues (see Figure 6.3). This again may reflect the younger age of women doctors or may be due to career interruption for childbirth.

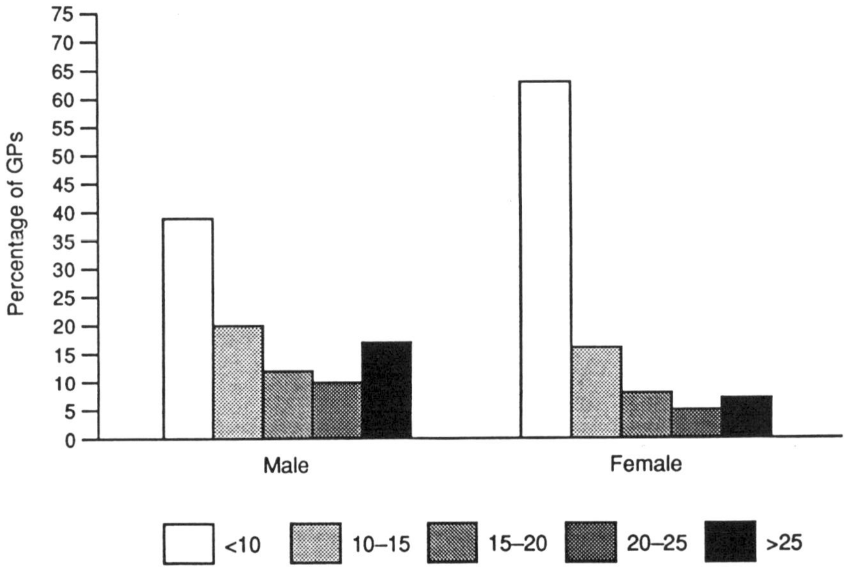

Figure 6.3. Years in general practice by gender

Practice location

Most of the GPs in the sample practiced in urban areas (66.8%) with only 33.1% practicing in rural and mixed areas (see Appendix 11). A higher percentage of female GPs (71.4%) practiced in urban areas than male GPs (65.9%).

Health behaviour outcomes

Smoking and drinking behaviour

Examining the total sample of the GPs, smoking was found to be very low (91.4% were non-smokers). This supports the finding that smoking has significantly reduced amongst doctors [194] probably because of their better knowledge of health. Because smokers tend to be lower down the socio-economic hierarchy (see Chapter 3) one would also expect professional groups such as doctors to indulge less in the habit. Large numbers (93.4%) of the sample continue to drink alcohol to some extent.

Generally, apart from isolated specific instances, it is the slow and gradual build up in consumption that is of interest, i.e. the 'heavy drinker' or the 'heavy smoker'. Whilst only a minority were shown to fall into such categories, some GPs tend to drink more heavily (5.4% had between 3 and 6 drinks daily and 0.4% had over 6 drinks daily). This is particularly significant in the light of the fact that these are probably conservative estimates, since individuals tend to under-report their drinking habits when self-reporting.

Although questionnaires are not the ideal method of enquiry for such a complex and emotive subject, the results that emerged indicated that this could well be a problem that deserves further and more specific investigation.

There was no significant differences between male and female GPs in terms of their smoking behaviour, but male GPs were found to consume significantly more alcohol than females. UK-trained GPs consumed significantly more alcohol than overseas-trained GPs, with no difference in smoking behaviour. Difference in drinking behaviour may be due to differences in the cultural background of overseas qualified GPs. There were no significant differences between principal GPs and trainee GPs in terms of either their drinking or smoking behaviour. Finally, there were no differences between rural practice GPs and urban practice GPs in terms of either drinking or smoking behaviour.

Stress outcomes

Mental health

Three scales of the Crown Crisp Experiential Index were used to measure levels of anxiety, depression and somatic anxiety among this group. Compared to national normative data, women GPs had significantly lower scores on free floating anxiety, depression and somatic anxiety. Male GPs, on the other hand, had significantly higher levels of free floating anxiety than the British normative male population (see Appendix 18). They showed no significant difference compared with male norms on depression but had significantly lower scores on the somatic anxiety scale (see Appendix 18). Women GPs appeared to have significantly increased levels of mental wellbeing whereas male GPs were more emotionally anxious but did not reflect this in psychosomatic complaints.

Job satisfaction

The highest levels of satisfaction were reported for the amount of responsibility, the freedom to choose methods of working and amount of variety in the job. This supports Cartwright and Anderson's findings [9] that GPs enjoy the diversity of their work and appreciate their freedom and independence. The lowest levels of satisfaction were reported for hours of work, recognition for good work, and the rate of pay (see Appendix 12). We found that women GPs were significantly more satisfied with their job than male GPs. This is an interesting finding in that women with professional jobs generally report greater levels of job satisfaction. Mawardi [84] reported "GPs as a group, scored next to least job satisfaction, paediatricians scored the lowest". She also added that 'many internists were unhappy because they handled too many minor illnesses and believed they served as GPs rather than main specialists'.

A significant difference emerged between UK-qualified GPs and overseas-qualified GPs, where the mean job satisfaction score was less for overseas-qualified GPs. This may be due to the unsatisfactory achievement of overseas-doctors in their career aspirations. Many of them come to the UK with the aim of benefiting from further training and gaining further professional qualifications, and then to return home highly qualified. Yet language difficulties, cultural differences and race discrimination may result in these objectives being blocked [262]. Their choice of general practice may be as a 'second-best' alternative to their preferred career choice. The doctor who has made a mistake by choosing a wrong career must live with it. The doctor who is trapped in the wrong job suffers from strain and becomes dissatisfied. In the words of an overseas-qualified GP from the interview sample:

> "Had I been able to achieve my ambitions, I would have become a specialist after passing my post-graduate medical examination. But here I am trapped in the wrong profession and just pushing myself in this job."

Rural GPs were more satisfied in their job than the urban practice GPs.

The authors' result supports the finding of Linn *et al.* [263] in their national study of physicians, that salary was one of the sources of job dissatisfaction. Many of the GPs in the interview sample felt underpaid and lacked prestige. One GP from the interview sample commented:

> "Our pay has fallen behind significantly in comparison to other professions. We are underpaid for the amount of responsibility we take for the society and our profession is lacking the prestige that we deserve, especially in those groups of people who try to use us as cheap labour."

Type A coronary prone behaviour

Type A coronary prone behaviour is characterised by a distinct sense of time urgency, restlessness, hostility, haste and extreme competitiveness and feelings of being under challenge of responsibility (Chapter 3). The distribution of Type A behaviour in the general population tends to be type A1, 10%; type A2, 40%; type B3, 40%; and type B4, 10% [146]. Type A1 signifies the most highly developed behaviour, and type B4 the most extreme type B behaviour [153]. GPs exhibit above-average levels of type A1 behaviour with 18.08% of respondents falling into type A1 category and 33.98% falling into type A2 category (see Appendix 13). Only 3.57% appeared in the type B4 category. It is obvious that the distribution of type A scores in the GP sample is positively skewed towards the higher end of this scale.

It was found that type A scores for overseas qualified GPs were significantly higher than for UK-qualified GPs. Male GPs reached a mean score of 93.09 which proves highly significant in relation to the senior male managers score of 69.0. Female GPs reach a mean score of 92.39 which again is highly significant in relation to the score for senior female managers of 73.3. When GPs scores are compared with those of police detectives the difference in scores is also highly significant (see Appendix 14).

We have already discussed that doctors appear to be compulsive individuals who are achievement orientated (Chapter 3). It was also found from Krackowski's [69] study that 100% of 100 physicians who were polled randomly declared themselves 'compulsive personalities'. Nelson [113] describes the physician as an 'ought to' person who takes pride in over production. These characteristics are in line with someone exhibiting high type A behaviour.

GPs with type A personality may organise their working day differently and may perceive stress in a more exaggerated fashion than GPs with type B personalities. Type A individuals are always deeply concerned with controlling their surroundings which results in damaging 'learned helplessness'. When they attempt to cope with non-controllable situations within a time limit it becomes difficult for them to manage without lowering standards. In this context it is worth mentioning a tragic loss of a GP due to suicide. Doctor X, 42, of Norfolk who took a drug overdose had set himself very high targets of achieving his goals. His wife told the inquest, "He set himself impossibly high tasks. He simply tried to do too much. He worked too hard and gave too much of himself". The coroner said "He was clearly a hardworking and very committed doctor – perhaps he was too committed". (General Practitioner, July 22, 1988).

If the majority of doctors exhibit type A personalities, there are certain important factors to be considered in relation to occupational stress. Firstly it is necessary to determine whether general practice as an occupation either attracts type A individuals or facilitates the development of type A behaviour in individuals. Type A individuals possess personality traits which actually facilitate self-selection into occupations that involve greater exposure to stressors [157]. Nevertheless, it was suggested by Frankenhauser [264] that occupational stressors can in fact encourage type A behaviour patterns.

Table 6.1 Job stressors identified by GPs: Factor analysis of stressors

Factor 1: Demands of the job and patients expectations (62.8% of variance)
- Fear of assault during night visits
- Visiting in extremely adverse weather conditions
- Adverse publicity by media
- Increased demands by patients and relatives for second opinion from hospital specialists
- No appreciation of your work by patients
- Worrying about patients' complaints
- Finding a locum
- Twenty-four hour responsibility for patients' lives
- Taking several samples in a short time
- Unrealistically high expectations by others of your role

Factor 2: Interruptions (10.6% of variance)
- Coping with phone calls during night and early morning
- Night calls
- Interruption of family life by telephone
- Emergency calls during surgery hours
- Home visits
- Dealing with problem patients
- Remaining alert when on call

Factor 3: Practice administration and routine medical (8.6% of variance)
- Hospital referrals and paperwork
- Conducting surgery
- Practice administration
- Arranging admission
- Working environment (surgery set-up)
- Time pressure

Factor 4: Home–work interface and social life (7.7% of variance)
- Demands of your job on family life
- Dividing time between spouse and patients
- Demands of your job on social life
- Lack of emotional support at home, especially from spouse

Factor 5: Dealing with death and dying (5.5% of variance)
- Daily contact with dying and chronically ill patients
- Dealing with terminally ill and their relatives

Factor 6: Medical responsibility for friends and relatives (4.4% of variance)
- Dealing with friends as patients
- Dealing with relatives as patients

Unfortunately, until type A questionnaires are administered to an appropriate sample of new medical entrants, trainee GPs and principal GPs, the question regarding type A behaviour in the general practice population will remain unanswered.

Stress vulnerability profiles

Potential sources of stress, identified by in-depth interviews (see Chapter 5), were rated on a 5-point scale and the 38 items were analysed to identify common stressor

Table 6.2. Factor analysis of the coping behaviour variables

Items	*Loadings*
Factor 1 – Seeking support (50.2% of variance)	
Talked to someone about how I was feeling	0.74
Talked to someone who could do something about the problem	0.59
Let my feelings out some way	0.48
Factor 2 – Denying (30.3% of variance)	
Didn't let it get to me; refusal to think about it too much	0.62
Went on as if nothing had happened	0.54
Factor 3 – Regretting (19.5% of variance)	
Blamed myself	0.54
Wished I could have changed what happened	0.54
Went over the problem again and again	0.48

Factor 1 – Seeking support
This factor consisted of responses to a group of three questions, i.e. 'talked to someone about how I was feeling', 'talked to someone who could do something about the problem' and 'let my feelings out some way'. In this case the individual is likely to externalise the problem some way, i.e. by talking to someone such as wife, husband, friend or colleague or asking for help.

Factor 2 – Denying
This factor is composed of two related responses in which the individual refused to think about it too much (didn't let it get to me) and 'went on as if nothing had happened'. It can be suggested that in this case the individual copes defensively by neglecting or denying that a problem exists.

Factor 3 – Regretting
These elements are identified within this area: 'blamed myself', 'wished I could have changed what happened' and 'went over the problem again and again'. In this case, it can be suggested that the respondents were employing a 'typical regret response'. In this response the problem is acknowledged by the individual but feelings of inability to cope and guilty feelings are present within the individual.

These factors are similar to those described by Hingley and Cooper (1986) [45].

themes or patterns. The items were grouped statistically into 6 factors or themes (see Table 6.1. Factor analysis was also performed on the coping variables which formed three alternative coping styles (see Table 6.2).

Figure 6.4 shows the stress vulnerability profiles of GPs most 'at risk' of showing symptoms of stress, i.e. mental ill health and alcohol consumption. These 'high risk' profiles were formulated by using step wise multiple regression analysis which relates independent and dependent variables in a way which takes interactive effects into account.

Mental ill health: 'high risk' profiles of GPs

The GP most 'at risk' in relation to mental ill health symptoms is someone who often adopts negative coping strategies (i.e. blamed themselves and wished they could have changed what happened, and went over the problem again and again) and who at work is subjected to high pressure associated with patients' expectations and demands on the job. In addition, unpredictable interruptions especially outside 'normal' working hours are the greatest source of stress. In this respect GPs are different from comparable groups; for many other groups the main sources of stress are overwork, both in terms of quantity and quality, role conflict and role ambiguity [58]. These factors do not appear to be particularly important for GPs. A cause of stress among GPs are unplanned and largely unpredictable events. The fourth predictor of mental ill health is 'work/home interface and social life'. It seems that the GP finds it difficult to adjust the time between home, work and social life. Again those GPs are more under stress who do not get emotional support from their spouses. 'Administration and routine medical' was also found to be a predictor of mental ill health. These work stressor factors seem to be more significant sources of stress, affecting mental well-being, among older GPs.

The profile of the 'high risk' male GP is that he is likely to be older and subjected to high pressure associated with patients' demands and expectations, interruptions, work/home conflict and administration (see Figure 6.4A). The profile of the 'high risk' mental illness-prone female GP is somewhat different. She is likely to be qualified overseas and adopts negative coping strategies to cope with stressors. She is also subjected to high pressure associated with work/home conflict, interruptions and administration (see Figure 6.4A). It is important to note that male GPs were affected more by the work-related aspects of the job, while female GPs were affected with the job interfering with their family life. There is evidence that conflicting demands from home and work can be very stressful. For example, Cooper [125] found that more and more married women are either divorcing, limiting their family size, or coping with both worlds at the expense of their physical and psychological health. The female GPs in this study were probably putting up with the conflict between work and home life at the expense of their mental health.

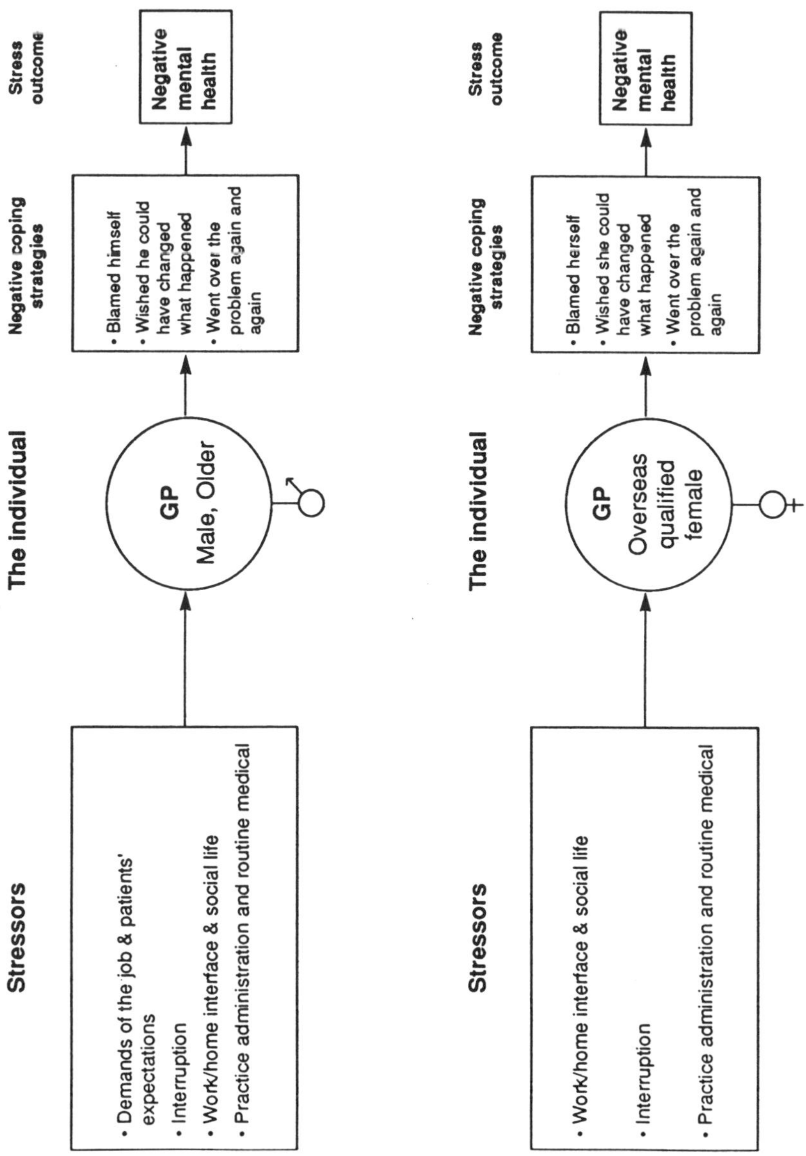

Figure 6.4A. Predictors of mental ill health in male and female GPs

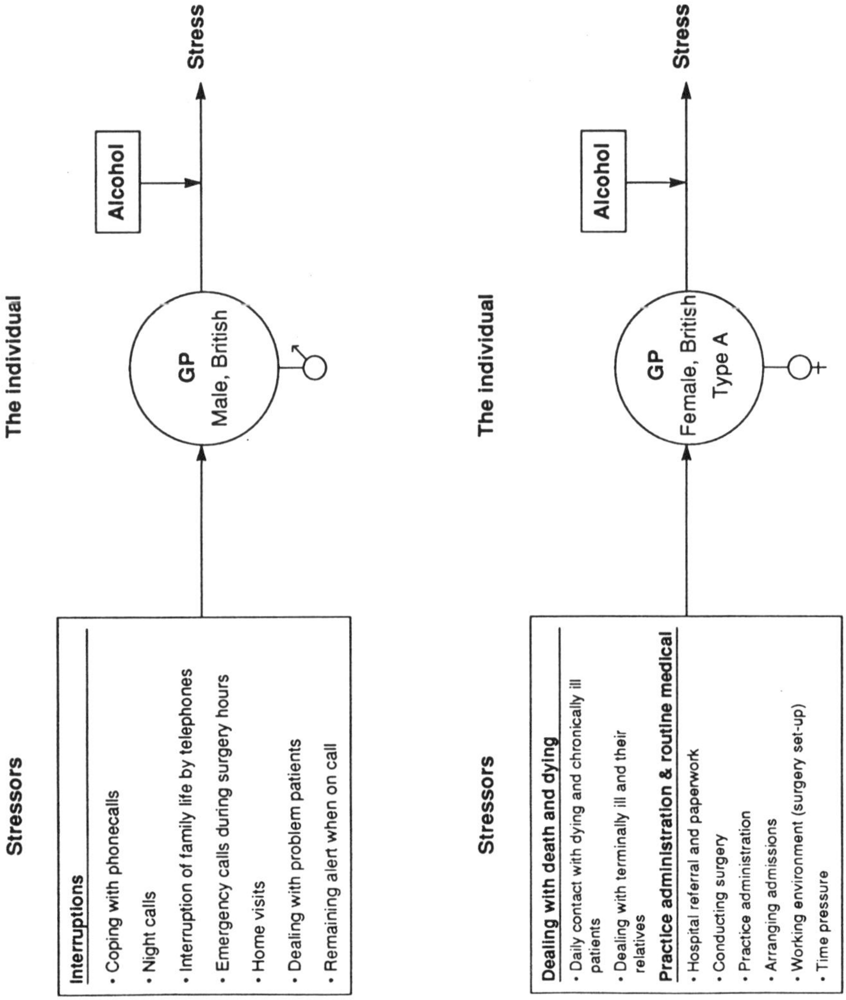

Figure 6.4B. Predictors of alcohol drinking in male and female GPs

In dealing with mental health subscales, it was found that five variables significantly predict anxiety in GPs. As was the case for overall mental health, 'negative' coping behaviour factor (regretting) is one of the important predictors of anxiety. It is interesting to note that GPs, whether male or female, who tend to exhibit type A behaviour pattern are most at risk of anxiety. Work/home conflict came as the most significant factor for female GPs whereas interruption was the most significant factor for male GPs.

In addition, another negative coping factor (denying) was one of the predictors of anxiety for female GPs. This can be interpreted that female GPs 'thought of the problem repeatedly' which is maladaptive in nature . In summary, it can be said that female GPs most at risk were the ones who tended to exhibit type A behaviour pattern in their life style and adapted 'negative' coping strategies.

GPs with somatic anxiety illness seem to be troubled by the same four work stressor factors, (i.e. demands of the job and patients' expectations; work/home interface and social life; practice administration and routine medical; and interruption) as in the case of overall mental health. Male GPs who are older suffer most from somatic anxiety when faced with the stress of work, whereas female GPs who exhibit type A behaviour pattern and qualified overseas suffer most from somatic anxiety when faced with the stress of work. The most significant predictor of somatic anxiety of female GPs was one of the negative coping factors (regretting). It is most likely that overseas qualified female GPs who have reflected a type A behaviour pattern in their life style, have more difficulty in balancing the workload between the family responsibility and their career and hence show greater incidence of psycho-somatic symptoms.

Again the same four stressor factors emerged as the predictors of depression for the whole sample and for male GPs. Older male GPs were most at risk, as was the case with somatic anxiety. For male GPs avoidance of seeking support and adoption of negative coping strategy emerge as significant predictors of depression. Male GPs who were depressed did not talk about their feelings or problems to someone who could do something about it. This is true of any depressive person; GPs are not superhumans.

The female GPs who were depressed thought about the event again and again. Only two stressor factors such as 'interruption' and 'work/home interface' are predictive of depression in the case of female GPs. However, it can be summarised that those women GPs who were depressed, were older, and used negative coping strategies to overcome work stress such as 'interruption' and 'home/work conflict'.

Job satisfaction: 'high risk' profiles of GPs

The GP most at risk in feeling high levels of job dissatisfaction is one who experiences high pressure due to stressors associated with the demands on the job, patients' expectations, work/home conflict and social life, interruption in the surgery and at home and administrative responsibility in the job. In addition 'gender' entered into the equation as one of the predictors of job satisfaction. This explains that male GPs were more dissatisfied in their job because of the presence of the above factors.

The same four stressor factors emerged in both the equations when the data was examined for male and female GPs. However, the most significant factor for female GPs was 'work/home interface and social life' while for male GPs, it was the 'demands on the job' and 'patients' expectation' factor. The highly dissatisfied female GP experiences high pressures from work/home conflict and not being able to maintain a good social life. Surprisingly, male GPs did not mind taking medical responsibility for friends and relatives whereas female GPs did.

Drinking: 'high risk' profiles of GPs

The male GP who drinks most alcohol is qualified in the UK and is interrupted less in the surgery or at home (see Figure 6.4B). The previous chapter showed that most of overseas qualified GPs do not drink at all. This may be due to their religious and cultural backgrounds. The female GP who drinks most has type A behaviour pattern, was qualified in the UK and was troubled with emotional aspects of the job and administrative responsibility in the surgery.

The popular view that dealing with the terminally ill and their relatives is an important source of occupational stress among GPs was not confirmed in this study. This aspect of the GPs job may, however, be implicated in a higher consumption of alcohol. This also suggests that there is some association between drinking behaviour and having to cope with chronically ill and dying patients, particularly for female GPs.

Smokers: 'high risk' profiles of GPs

The result was not significant for either male or female GPs.

Chapter 7 – VARIATIONS BETWEEN GENERAL PRACTITIONERS

In this chapter the significant differences between GPs by gender, practice type, job title, practice location and place of qualification in response to work stressors are considered.

Are women doctors more stressed than men?

The mean scores for female GPs were significantly higher than the male GPs on the following stressors (see Appendix 21): practice administration, coping with numerous journals and newsletters, daily contact with dying and chronically ill patients, fear of assault during night visits, dealing with the terminally ill and their relatives, dealing with friends and relatives as patients, coping with new technology, partner on holiday, finding a locum and visiting in extremely adverse weather conditions.

Dealing with death and chronic illness

Daily contact with dying and chronically ill patients emerged as a clear identifiable area of stress for female GPs. Not surprisingly, the respondents found that caring for life in the face of death, the chronically ill and terminally ill is fundamentally threatening to a human being who is herself vulnerable to the illness and death she is caring for. Dealing with the dying and chronically ill produced feelings of inadequacy and powerlessness. One female GP (interview sample) commented:

> "I feel very bad when I know that the patient is dying but he does not accept it. Contact with these kind of patients gives me anxiety which eventually leads to complete emotional exhaustion. I talk it over with my husband when I go home, who himself is a doctor. He seems to be unmoved with these kind of emotional aspects, advises me that I shouldn't be attached to a patient whose death is inevitable."

The mean stressor score for female GPs in response to 'dealing with terminally ill and their relatives' was higher than for male GPs. It is a big dilemma for a GP attending a terminally ill patient whether to break the bad news which may devastate his emotional state or just be pleasant by hiding the real diagnosis from him. It is even worse in the case of female GPs. One female GP commented:

> "I find it extremely difficult to tell the true diagnosis to a patient whom I've known very well for many years who is suffering from an incurable disease. In

> one way I try to keep him happy by hiding the facts away from him but on the other hand it makes me feel guilty for not telling the truth. It is even worse during his dying moments."

Dealing with friends and relatives as patients

The mean stressor scores for 'dealing with friends and relatives as patients', were significantly higher for women GPs. As a woman GP illustrated:

> "One evening one of my aunties complained of discomfort in her chest while I was in her house. She is known to have similar problems to anxiety. When my uncle requested me to examine her, I simply advised him to get in touch with their own doctor as I felt my diagnosis may be biased and I did not want to get the blame in case her symptoms were due to some pathological reasons."

From the above comments it can be assumed that GPs on the whole do not like dealing with friends and relatives and in the case of women, they may be more sensitive to emotional matters. This may be the reason why female GPs find it more stressful to deal with friends and relatives as patients than the male GPs.

Coping with new technology

'Coping with new technology' was a significantly greater stressor for women GPs. This may be a result of early sexual stereotyping. In the interview sample GPs expressed a need for continuing education and training to keep abreast with new technology especially for those women GPs who return to their profession after maternity leave or after raising children for a number of years. These women found themselves de-skilled and out of touch.

Holidays and locums

Female GPs reported higher mean stressor scores in response to 'partner on holiday' and 'finding a locum' compared to their male colleagues. Most women doctors tend to work in partnerships where all their colleagues were men [261] and they often choose to work part-time to suit their family and social commitment (as shown in the interview sample). But the problem arises that when a full-time partner goes away on holiday the part-time woman GP is burdened with the problem of managing the surgery and finding a locum. On the other hand for male GPs this is not a major problem as they are more used to working full-time and cover their colleagues during their absence.

Fear of assault

The female GPs showed more stress for 'fear of assault during night visits' than the male GPs. In general, women are more prone to physical attack by nature of their gender and their lesser ability to defend themselves. It is not surprising that most of the women respondents showed greater pressure for 'fear of assaults' during night visits. A young woman GP said:

> "I am scared to do visits in the late evenings. I try to avoid as much as I can to do night visits by advising patients on the telephone. If it becomes absolutely necessary to visit I use the deputising service even if I have to pay."

Visiting in bad weather

Women GPs reported higher mean stressor scores than their male counterparts in response to 'visiting in extremely adverse weather conditions'. It has been found that women GPs use more deputising services and in general spend fewer nights 'on call' than male GPs [9]. As a result they are less used for visiting patients in adverse weather conditions. One woman GP from the interview sample commented:

> "Sometimes patients request a visit during bad weather only because they do not like to come to the surgery in such bad weather conditions. They never think of the doctor's feelings should be exactly like their own but unfortunately I have to do the visit even if I hate it."

Coping with keeping up-to-date

Compared to males, female GPs reported greater stress associated with 'coping with numerous journals and newsletters'. Like many other professions education does not stop at the end of the formal training period in general practice. Ideally, it continues throughout the professional career of the GP. Changes in knowledge, technique and treatment require the GP to keep up-to-date with developments. However, there are now around 800 English language medical journals covering every topic and speciality and the GP cannot possibly hope to cover even a fraction of them. In the case of women GPs, they may have the added responsibility of caring for the family and have less time to spare to go through large numbers of medical newsletters and journals. As one woman doctor in our interview sample put it:

> "After the end of the surgery I rush home to see my children. I have hardly any time to open the vast number of medical journals that come through the post. But I realise how much I miss out on recent developments. It is very embarrassing when my partners discuss new treatments and techniques and I am unable to take part in it."

Do group practice GPs report more stress than solo practice GPs?

Group practice GPs reported significantly greater pressure on 14 stressors than single-handed GPs (see Appendix 17). Single-handed GPs, however, were more stressed by only five different stressors.

The mean pressure score for group practice GPs on practice administration and conflict with partners were significantly higher than for single-handed GPs. This may be due to the management of large numbers of ancillary staff, large volume of accounts, maintenance of a satisfactory standard of record system, storage of data and stock control in group practices. In the case of single-handed practices there are a limited number of ancillary staff to manage and no question of conflict with partners. It was found that a larger number of single-handed practitioners preferred to be in District Health Authority Health Centres [261], where the staff and cleaners are appointed by the health authority. This reduces the practising GPs' burden on practice administration.

GPs in group practices show a higher degree of concern during partner's (partners') holidays. In this case, they are obliged to cover for their colleagues during their absence and this increases workload and imposes additional responsibility. The single-handed practice GPs usually fix a locum or make arrangements with neighbouring colleagues for holiday cover.

There was a significant difference on 'time pressure' between the two groups, group practice GPs showing more pressure than solo practice GPs. In a group practice much time may be taken up by co-ordination, communication and organisation between the doctors and the staff, including the practice manager. It is also time consuming to discuss patient care with the members of the primary health care team (i.e. attached nurses, practice nurses, practice managers, etc.). Possibly single-handed GPs do not get involved or committed as much to many health care activities. Therefore there is less time pressure in this context. This was summed up by one GP in the interview sample:

> "We have too many bloody meetings: partnership meetings, clinical meetings, medical film shows, primary health care team meetings, etc. Too many people talk about too many things but achieve too little. In our practice meetings my senior partner's words are always taken as gospel. All these meetings are too time consuming and a big waste as well."

The mean scores for 'night calls', 'dealing with problem patients', 'demands of job on family life', 'coping with phone calls during night and early morning' and 'emergency calls during surgery hours' are high for both single-handed and group practice GPs but group practice GPs showed significantly higher pressure than solo practice GPs. On the basis of these results, however, the authors are unwilling to speculate on the reason. Further in-depth research into activities of solo and group practices is required in order to establish the reason.

Although the mean scores for the following stressors: 'coping with numerous journals and newsletters', 'conducting surgery', 'home visits', 'remaining alert when on call', and 'dealing with friends as patients' were not very high for the two groups of GPs, there was a significant difference between them. Here again group practice GPs showed higher mean response to the above stressors. There is some anecdotal evidence that some junior partners have been frustrated by the attitude of their more traditional senior partners and had left the partnership to take up solo practices which provided opportunities for innovation and transformation. For a young, enthusiastic and dynamic ambitious GP, a solo practice can be a source of personal satisfaction. Often anecdotal evidence suggests that the junior partner often shouldered a heavier workload of surgery consultations, home visits and commitments, while the senior partner retained power solely in his hands.

'Finding a locum' shows significantly higher mean response for the single-handed GP. A single-handed GP is well acquainted with his patients and has a personal bonding with them. He may be worried that a locum may not provide the same quality of care to his patients and will break the continuity of care. It may also not be possible to find a locum readily available to suit his timings.

Single-handed GPs showed significantly higher pressure on the stressor: '24 hours responsibility for patients lives'. A single-handed GP committed to 24 hours cover for his patients finds it strenuous as he has no one else with whom to share his workload. One of the single-handed GPs in the interview sample commented:

> "It is alright for doctors who are in group practices to relax and enjoy but for me I am 24 hours on call and can't go anywhere, even to my next-door neighbour, without carrying the bleep."

Wilkin *et al.* [261] found that among all single-handed GPs, 28% claimed regularly to spend some part of every weekend on call, and 32% claimed to be on call for some part of every week night. Only 3% and 2% respectively of GPs in group practices did so since they were able to share the burden among partners. The commitment of the isolated GP was in fact even greater than these figures suggest; 45% were on call every weekend and 52% every weekday night. This contrasts sharply with the 13% and 26% of their single-handed colleagues who worked alongside other doctors. The same pattern was evident with respect to holidays so that isolated doctors took an average of 3 weeks per year, compared with 5 weeks for both other single-handed and partnered GPs.

It appears from the respondents that single-handed GPs find it more stressful to drive in adverse weather conditions to do their visits than the group practice GPs. Possibly, a single-handed GP is more apprehensive of immediate breakdown in snowy and frosty weather when he has no colleagues to offer him help in doing his visits. One single-handed GP in the interviews said:

> "The GPs in group practice at least have an option of asking for help from their colleagues in cases of emergency but in my case, I have to wait for AA rescue service."

Again, in the area of 'adverse publicity in the press', the GPs in solo practices reported significantly more pressure than GPs in group practices. This is perhaps due to the fact that the solo GP has no colleagues to share the responsibility and give him moral support in difficult situations unlike as in group practices where a second opinion from colleagues can be obtained in doubtful situations. There remains the anxiety of being exploited and exposed by his own patients, but most of all 'adverse publicity in the press' remains one of the most stressful factors.

Although the mean scores on 'lack of emotional support from spouse' are not very high for both the groups, there is still a significant difference between these two groups, in that single-handed GPs showed more pressure than the group practice GPs. Probably single-handed GPs are on call more nights during the week which keeps them away from home for considerably longer hours.

Are trainees in better shape than principals?

Trainees scored significantly higher than the principals in seven questions (see Appendix 16). Principal GPs showed more pressure than the trainees in only one variable: 'conflict with partners in a group practice'.

Trainees come from the hospital service straight into general practice which represent a very different organisation. The trainee GP without much experience in general practice is very likely to experience more stress than the principal GPs. They never had to do any home visits in their hospital career; when they realise that seeing patients in their home at any time and in any weather condition is a part of their job, they may feel more stressed than the principals.

In comparison to principal GPs trainee GPs felt it more stressful to collect several samples in a limited period because of their lack of skills, technique and shortage of time (i.e. when the patients have been allocated a limited time period during which a decision has to be taken). This may be related to the fact that doctors in hospitals do not have to take the samples themselves as there are technicians and nurses to do such jobs. As one of the trainee GPs in the interview sample said:

> "You've got to do everything on your own here, there are no technicians or nurses to do these simple jobs for you. I could utilise this time in a better way."

Probably a major part of their allocated time for each patient is taken up by taking samples and less or no time is left for the clinical management of that patient. Due to this shortage of time they feel under pressure.

Mean pressure scores for 'dealing with terminally ill and their relatives' were higher for trainees compared to principals. A young trainee GP said during the interviews:

> "When a terminally ill patient is admitted to hospital the doctor deals with the medical problem but the physical tender loving care is left to the nursing and ancillary staff. Here, I am being asked to arrange a commode, bed pan, district nurse, health visitor, night sitter and so on. I find dealing with demanding

relatives is more of a problem than dealing with the patient."

As described earlier trainee GPs do not have much practical experience in general practice. They have clinical training in hospital but in general practice treating a terminally ill patient requires skills in social as well as clinical fields.

Trainees showed more pressure than the principal GPs in 'examining patients of the opposite sex'. Trainees are used to examining patients of the opposite sex in hospital when a chaperone is readily available, whereas not many practices have nurses employed to do such jobs. Although it is possible to call one of the other staff to attend as a chaperone, because of the shortage of time they frequently have to go ahead with the examination alone. One of the male trainee GPs in the interview sample said:

"The younger the woman patient the more I feel awkward to examine her."

Principal GPs reported greater mean pressure scores compared to trainee GPs on 'conflict with partners in a group practice'. Obviously as the trainee GP is normally working only for either 6 or 12 months as an employee, employed by his trainer, he does not have any links with the partnership. In the case of principal GPs, partners have to work together even if there are conflicting disagreements in many areas. Stress might occur as either some of the partners are forced to compromise in certain matters with their colleagues even if it is against their wish or when they fail to compromise but continue working together.

Are overseas doctors more under stress?

It was found that there were significant differences between overseas and UK-qualified GPs on 23 variables (see Appendix 19). Of these 23 variables, overseas-qualified doctors found 17 variables to be of significantly higher pressure than UK-qualified doctors.

The average pressure score for overseas GPs in response to the statement 'lack of emotional support from spouse' was significantly higher than for UK-qualified GPs. Spouses of overseas qualified GPs often have the disadvantage of not having their parents or close relations in this country. Their husbands are the main and often the only social support to their families. The busy doctor deprives his spouse of her share of attention and care because of his out-of-hours commitments. In one study, Elliot [265] found that the doctors' heavy workload meant that their wives were taking on the role of father/husband as well as their own wife/mother role, and were exhausted and overwhelmed by the dual responsibility. This heavy burden on doctors' wives reflects in lack of emotional support for their husbands.

The mean pressure scores for both UK- and overseas-qualified GPs in response to 'worrying about patients complaints' was quite high. However, the mean pressure scores for overseas-qualified GPs was significantly higher than UK-qualified GPs. Also the mean pressure score for 'adverse publicity in the press' was significantly higher for overseas-qualified GPs, compared to UK-qualified GPs. As increasing numbers of cases of complaints about doctors are brought to the courts, this must be causing intense stress among the GPs, as they are the first line of patient contact. Overseas doctors in particular take this seriously as they may think they are more prone to such complaints because of prejudice and discrimination. This was highlighted by one of the overseas GPs we interviewed:

> "However good I am, one cannot remove prejudice and racial discrimination from people's minds. I have to be very careful of what I do because a slight error might bring my name on the front page of the local newspaper. No one will appreciate your good work but a minute mistake will take you to hell."

Average pressure scores for '24 hour responsibility for patients lives' was significantly higher for overseas-qualified GPs than UK-qualified GPs. Unlike in the UK, in many of the countries from which they came doctors do not have to bear 24 hour responsibility for their patients lives. Thus the overseas qualified doctors may not find it easy to cope with the arrangements of the NHS in this country, where they have to take responsibility day and night for their patients.

'No appreciation of your work by patients' was associated with higher levels of pressure by overseas-qualified GPs. In general, both groups of doctors felt that their job is not appreciated by their patients but it is felt more by overseas doctors. It could be assumed that the overseas doctors' origin and pride of social standing makes them expect to gain prestige and appreciation from the people they care for but the absence of this makes them feel stressful.

'Increased demand by patients and relatives for a second opinion from hospital specialists' was a significantly greater stressor for overseas-qualified GPs than UK-qualified GPs. There are greater demands by the patients and their relatives on their GPs to refer them to hospital specialists for a second opinion even on simple matters. Perhaps the overseas-qualified GPs are not keen to refer such trivial cases to the hospital but on the other hand are worried of being accused by their patients of negligence.

'Dealing with the terminally ill and their relatives' yielded significantly higher mean scores from overseas-qualified doctors as well. Social structure in many overseas countries is totally different to the UK, especially in Asian countries where members of the family tend to live together and the elderly and the sick are cared for by other family members. Doctors qualified in such countries may not be used to the high demands of relatives of the terminally ill patients in the UK where the relatives themselves tend to take little or no responsibility. In this context one overseas GP in our interview sample commented:

> "I find people always produce excuses when they are asked to care for a terminally ill relative especially those who demand help from the doctors and other NHS services. Some of them are more keen in finding what is in the will than the therapy and care of the ill. If the relations would be prepared to accept at least a little responsibility the doctors' burden would be greatly reduced."

'Coping with new technology' and 'taking several samples in a short time' were associated with higher levels of pressure by overseas- than UK-qualified GPs. It is likely that GPs qualified abroad will have been trained in more traditional ways with less access to the modern technology such as ECG, vitalograph, sonicaid and computers to which they are exposed in the UK. For the latter item it can be suggested overseas-qualified doctors give more importance to clinical examination and depend on less laboratory investigation.

Mean pressure scores for overseas- and UK-qualified GPs were both low in response to 'examining patients of the opposite sex'. For a doctor, probing into the private parts of patients of the opposite sex is a part of physical examination but unfortunately may lead to complaints against doctors of malhandling during such examinations. Overseas doctors may find themselves at a disadvantage because of their ethnic origin. As one overseas GP commented during the interviews:

> "I try to be careful before examining a woman patient on her own. I always ask my receptionist to be there while examining. Some women with discriminative attitudes may find it easy to lodge a complaint that she has been sexually malhandled during examination without any real truth in it."

'Unrealistically high expectations by others of your role' and 'taking work home' were associated with higher levels of pressure by overseas doctors. It is worth noting a few comments made by overseas doctors during the interviews in relation to the former stressor:

> "In my country when a doctor goes to visit a patient the relation would come to the door step and greet him, carry his bag inside. But here I go to visit a patient sometimes I am asked to go to the chemist and fetch the medicine for the patient who lives alone and does not expect her son to come and get medicine until the next day."

> "The most annoying thing I find when patients expect me to take their urine, blood sample, and throat swab etc. to the local path lab. For example, one day a patient said to me 'I haven't got my car today, can you take the sample to the path lab for me?' I said, 'I am sorry but I don't run a taxi service'. I think they are not only expecting unrealistic things from us but simply using us."

In addition, two significant differences between overseas-qualified GPs and UK-qualified GPs were identified in relation to visiting patients. Overseas doctors were more likely to feel pressure as a consequence of 'visiting in adverse weather conditions' and as a result of 'fear of assault during night visits'. These differences suggest that overseas-qualified GPs experience greater difficulty in coping with adverse weather conditions and night visits. Possibly, they were not exposed to these conditions before coming to this country.

UK-qualified GPs found six different work stressors as significantly more stressful than the overseas-qualified GPs: 'conducting a surgery', 'dealing with problem patients', 'practice administration', 'emergency calls during surgery hours', 'demands of the job on family life' and 'time pressure'.

The most striking finding is that the UK-qualified GPs reported a much higher incidence of pressure arising from 'emergency calls during surgery hours', 'dealing with problem patients', and 'demands of job on family life'. In keeping with the findings for the main sample, these variables were most frequently reported as sources of stress by both the groups. UK-qualified GPs, however, expressed a relatively greater concern about 'practice administration' and 'conducting surgery' than did overseas-qualified GPs.

Are urban GPs more under stress?

There were significant differences between rural and urban practice GPs on 14 variables (see Appendix 20). Of these, urban practice GPs found 9 variables to be of significantly higher pressure than rural practice GPs. Although night call is a major stressor for both urban and rural GPs the former group suffer from it more. The reason may be due to the concentration of the socially disadvantaged and to people with more psychological problems in urban areas. Wilkin *et al.* [261] stated that the "inner city practice generates more work for the doctor than practising in an affluent suberb". Although the mean pressure scores are not very high for the stressor 'fear of assault during night visits' urban practice GPs showed significantly higher pressure than their rural practice counterparts.

Mean pressure scores for 'unrealistically high expectation by others of your role' however, was significantly higher for urban practice GPs compared to rural practice GPs. 'Adverse publicity in the press', 'worrying about patients complaints' and 'increased demands by patients and relatives for second opinion from the hospital specialist' were associated with higher levels of pressure by urban than rural practice GPs.

Rural GPs showed greater stress on 'coping with phone calls during the night and early morning', 'interruption of family life by telephone', 'demands of job on social life' and 'hospital referrals and paper work' than urban practice GPs. Not many rural areas have deputising services available; GPs practising in these areas are often on-call 24 hours. This means more interruptions by telephone at night and early morning and thus more interruptions of family and social life. Urban GPs usually have the option of passing on their responsibilities to deputising services.

Chapter 8 – STRESS MANAGEMENT AND GENERAL PRACTITIONERS

So far we have presented a detailed analysis and discussion of the qualitative and quantitative results of the study. It is the purpose of this chapter to draw together all the findings from the research and suggest some stress management and coping strategies. Also this chapter briefly mentions our post-contract qualitative study.

What can be done?

It seems that general practice is generally recognised as being a very demanding profession and stress has become an almost inevitable occupational hazard. The role of the doctor in society is 'to function at the maximum level of competence at all times' [266]. Taking 24 hour responsibility for patients who are ill and in crisis means that general practice will always be a potentially high stress profession and, for these reasons it is all the more important to identify the stressors involved (both at the individual and the organisational level) and to minimise the pressures by taking appropriate action.

Six broad sources of stress are identified in our study and Figure 8.1 shows how the outcome is a direct response of a GP's perception of the sources of stress and his skills in coping with them. Figures 8.2 and 8.3 show the effect of adapting positive and negative coping strategies in the workplace.

Demands of the job

Our study reveals that the GPs mental well-being and job satisfaction are affected by the following stress factors: 'demands of the job and patients' expectations', 'practice administration and routine medical', 'work/home interface and social life' and 'interruptions'. GPs are not satisfied with their job because of the demands of the job and lack of appreciation by the patients.

Patients' expectations have increased many fold and for some their 'wants' are more than their 'needs'. GPs could consider initiating patient participation groups where the patients learn how to share responsibility on health matters. Regular meetings will acquaint them with the GP's work pattern, workload and job demands. The expectation of patients can be reduced by increasing understanding and discussion between the doctor and the patients in such groups. Such participation may help to avert confrontation and litigation.

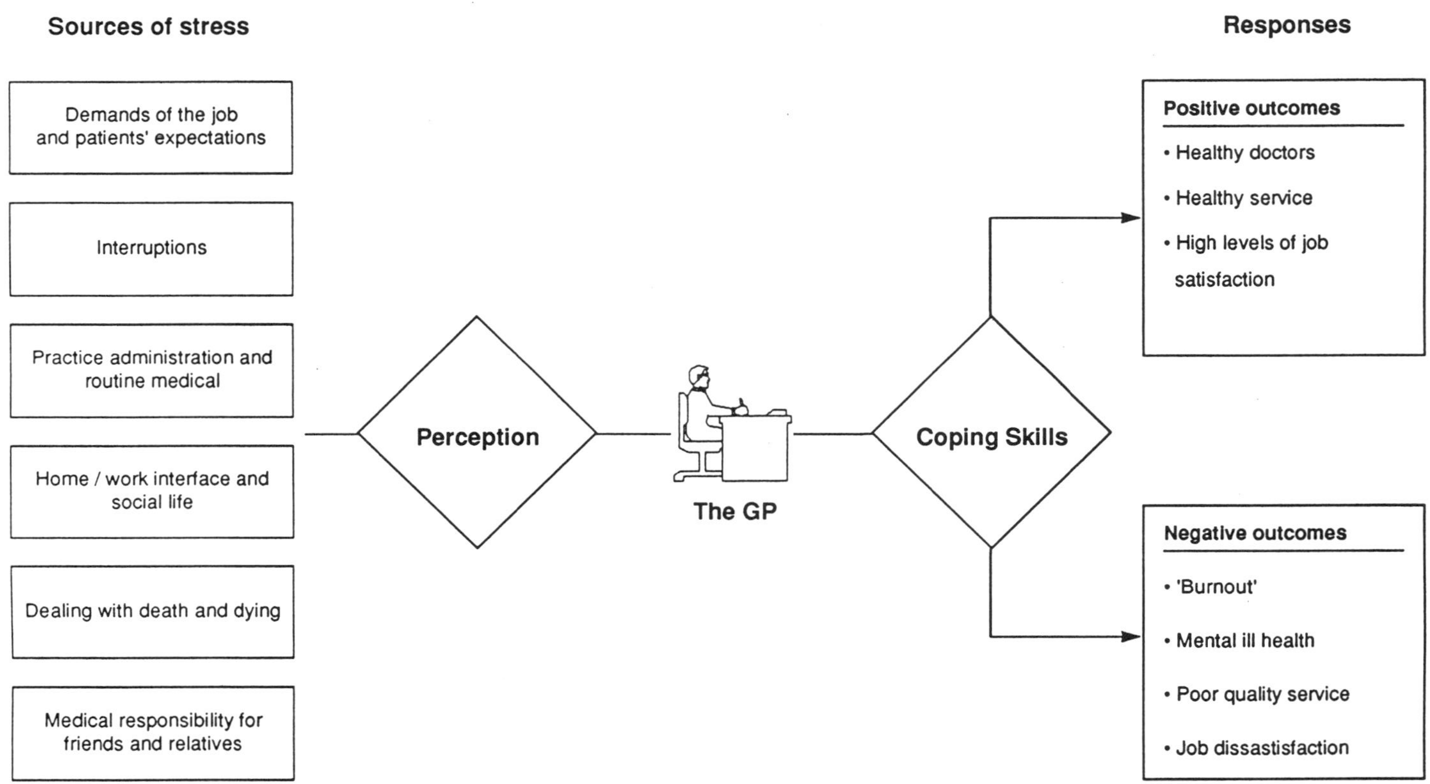

Figure 8.1.The six broad sources of stress identified in our study showing how the outcome is a direct response of a GP's perception of the sources of stress and his skill in coping with them

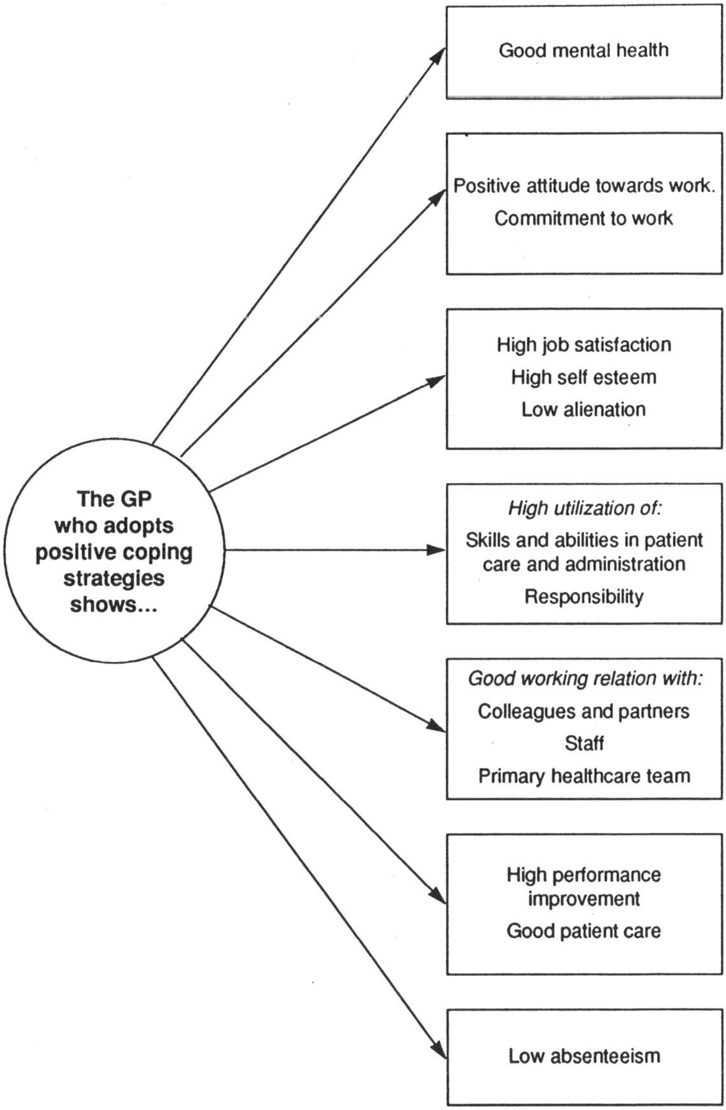

Figure 8.2. The effect of adapting positive coping strategies in the workplace

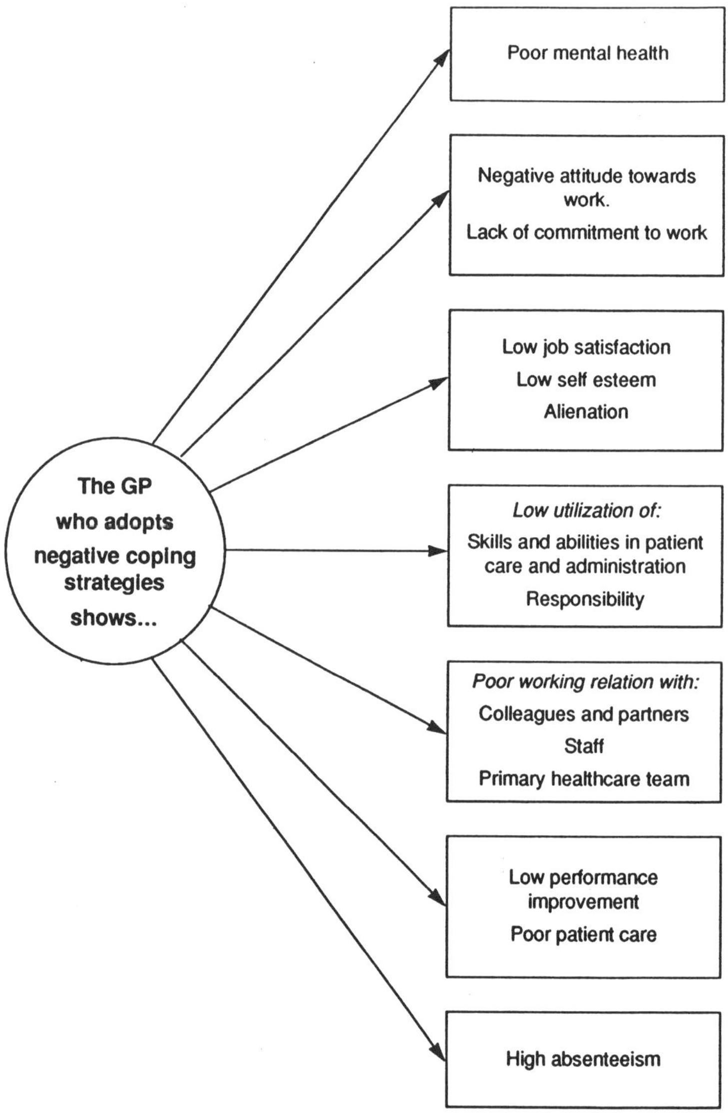

Figure 8.3. The effect of adapting negative coping strategies in the workplace

A practice nurse can ease the burdens of the doctor by treating minor ailments and also directing the patients to the appropriate authorities (i.e. social services, health visitor, district nurse, etc.) for non-medical help. Taking samples can also be delegated to a practice nurse. Psychosocial problems can be dealt with by employing a counsellor. Our interviews found that a large proportion of consultations were for non-medical problems which GPs did not enjoy dealing with due to time pressures. In a study in Bristol, Hudson [267] found that only 53% of patients attended the surgery for purely physical problems, 27% with psychiatric or psychological problems, 16% with social problems and 4% attended for trivial reasons. This raises the question of how GPs cope when nearly half of their patients attend the surgery with underlying social and psychological problems. Some GPs say the answer lies in the prescription pad and the use of psychotropic drugs. Gravelle [268] found that psychotropic drugs account for about 15% of all drug prescriptions and cost about one-fifth of the annual NHS expenditure on drugs. Mitchell [269] revealed that 1 in 50 of the adult population take tranquilizers permanently. This suggests that prescription of such drugs are often inappropriate, ineffective and unnecessary. Such action does not necessarily imply that doctors have been irresponsible in prescribing such drugs; considering the pressure that they are under in our stressful western society what alternatives do they have? There are only a very small number of clinical psychologists based at local hospitals to whom GPs can refer their patients; it would prove impossible to refer nearly half their patients to psychologists for specialist counselling.

GPs feel that they are inadequately trained to cope with the nonmedical problems encountered within general practice. As one GP has said:

> "I let the patient talk for a few minutes when I realise that their problem is not physical. Then I become aware that time is getting on, so I start writing a prescription. Patients always know that a prescription is the termination of a consultation and automatically stop talking." [267]

GPs may realise that it is not always easy to counsel a patient within a 5–10 minutes appointment and should recognise substantial advantages of using a qualified counsellor or counselling psychologist in these cases. Perhaps the government can be persuaded to recognise the need to establish employed qualified counsellors within all the major surgeries on a nation wide basis and make funds available to the FHSAs for reimbursement by GPs for their counsellors. If this concept is not accepted by the government, then GPs can substantially reduce their workload by employing a counsellor at their own expense; a number of practices could perhaps join together to employ a counsellor and share the costs.

Interruptions

Interruption of any kind is one of the major factors of stress in general practice. Its existence is inevitable but some steps may be taken to deal with it. Telephone interruptions during surgery hours can be unpleasant, annoying and frustrating especially while the GP is deeply involved in consultation with the patients. This can be avoided by instructing the staff to advise the caller that the doctor is busy in the surgery and he/she should ring later after the surgery hours. In very urgent cases the call may be put on 'hold' until after the end of the consultation which is usually indicated by the doctor asking to see the next patient. The GP may make himself available to receive routine telephone calls at a certain time of the day only, ideally after the end of the surgery. Patients have to be informed about this policy through practice leaflets and/or posters in the waiting room. For any other important telephone calls the caller should be told that the doctor is busy with a patient and he may leave his telephone number so that the doctor can return his call as soon as he is free. In group practices the working pattern for the doctors can be organised in such a way that one of the partners be available to deal with telephone calls and emergencies. The final policy needs to be tailored to the preferences of the doctors involved. It can be very helpful to make a time log to get some idea of the size of the interruption:

Day/Date	Source of interruption	Time taken	Reason	Urgency
Mon 1/2/93	Telephone (partner)	5 minutes	Problem patient	Low

The following points may help GPs in dealing with interruptions:

1. Specify your time of availability. Your interrupter may not have been aware of when you are available for general consultation and advice.

2. Give your interrupter an alternative. Tell people when you will next be free by giving a specific time range.

3. Tell your colleagues when you don't want to be interrupted, such as during consultations.

4. Give a time limit to how long you can spare, politely – 'I'm very busy but I can give you 2 minutes now'.

5. Ask the interrupter if the matter is urgent and has to be dealt with instantly and, if not, ask him or her to wait until you are free.

6. Use various techniques to cut short interruptions: glance at your watch, stand up (or remain standing), ask what the problem is.

7. Handle interrupters fairly – they are less likely to come back again; ensure that you give your full attention and the help that is needed.

8. Be brief and to the point on the telephone.

9. At home, if you have important work to do, agree a time when your family will not interrupt you and in return promise to spend time with them when your work is completed.

While on call the GP can take advantage of a modern telephone answering machine especially while having his meal. GPs can also choose to instruct the deputising service to hold on to non-urgent calls for a certain length of time. They may consider using modern radio pagers which can store several messages so that they can be dealt with later on. Urgent calls, however, will still need immediate action. For a peaceful and quiet night calls can be passed on to deputising services so that GPs can have a good rest and function efficiently the next morning. Monday morning surgeries could be avoided following a weekend on call. Several practices can organise a larger rota where the doctors will be on call less frequently. The familiar two hour evening surgery is usually highly pressurising when the GP is tired towards the end of the day. The appointments for these surgeries could be reduced to one hour only. Realistic time management would reduce the stress caused by frequent unnecessary interruptions.

The number of home visits can be reduced by offering an efficient appointment system with a short waiting time which in turn will reduce workload. Unnecessary requests for home visits can be reduced by educating the patients; patients should be encouraged to come to the surgery rather than receiving home visits. It may be better to have a 10-minute appointment system for each patient. Some GPs say that 5-minute appointments are not long enough to practice adequate medicine, and does not give enough time to complete forms, dictate letters, fit in emergencies and look at the medical records for the next patient. However, interruption is an integral part of general practice and the GP must learn how to cope with it through training at medical school as well as during vocational training.

Administration

Administration is one of the major stressors for GPs that ultimately affects their mental health and job satisfaction. By employing a trained practice manager a large load of their administrative burdens can be relieved. The practice manager can take charge of organising the doctors, staff, surgery timings, appointment system, staff wages, holidays, arranging locums, advertising and interviewing new staff, regular inspection to ensure maintenance of premises, arranging practice meetings, liaising with FHSA and health authorities, preparing annual reports, business plans and other reports as necessary, and general finance. Figure 8.4 shows a brief explanation of coping with the administrative and other problems of general practice.

GPs need to consider employing adequate staff to do all the relevant paperwork for the efficient functioning of the practice. We suggest that practices have a firm policy for everyone to follow and regular practice meetings should be held to resolve differences on administration, problems between partners and staff and to plan future strategies. GPs themselves should attend managerial training courses. Medical schools can help by introducing adequate training in administration. The new contract has increased administrative workload and pressures considerably [64]. GPs will have to acquire accountancy skills and administrative skills to cope with the increased workload

Home/work conflict

The conflicting demands of home and work affects the mental health and job satisfaction of GPs. The GP may fail to realise the importance of his companionship with the family by becoming a workaholic. Equal importance needs to be given to family life as much as to the job. Couples need to have their own time to spend together to express their feelings and emotions and discover ways to sort out any problem that may have arisen either at work or at home.

Doctors who are unable to develop their family life to the extent of being open and expressive about their feelings and desires at home will find that when they have a problem at work it is difficult for them to express these at home. Similar problems occur with doctors who have not developed friendship or other sorts of ties such that they can seek to express these in the supportive environment of friendship. In some cases the level of friendship is such that openness and trust is at a very limited level. It is advisable for him to make himself available to his family by taking time off and perhaps develop time management skill in order to apportion his time to work and to his family. This may be achieved by organising weekend rotas with colleagues, taking regular holidays and nights out.

Coping strategies

It was of little surprise to us to discover the strong association between mental ill health and negative coping strategies of GPs because mental and/or physical ill health can develop when either coping mechanisms are insufficient to relieve the load, or when the coping process continues over such a long period of time that the body or mind becomes exhausted. GPs internalise their feelings instead of dealing directly with them. Successful coping leads to health and well-being. It is advisable for GPs to use positive coping strategies rather than negative ones (Figures 8.2 and 8.3).

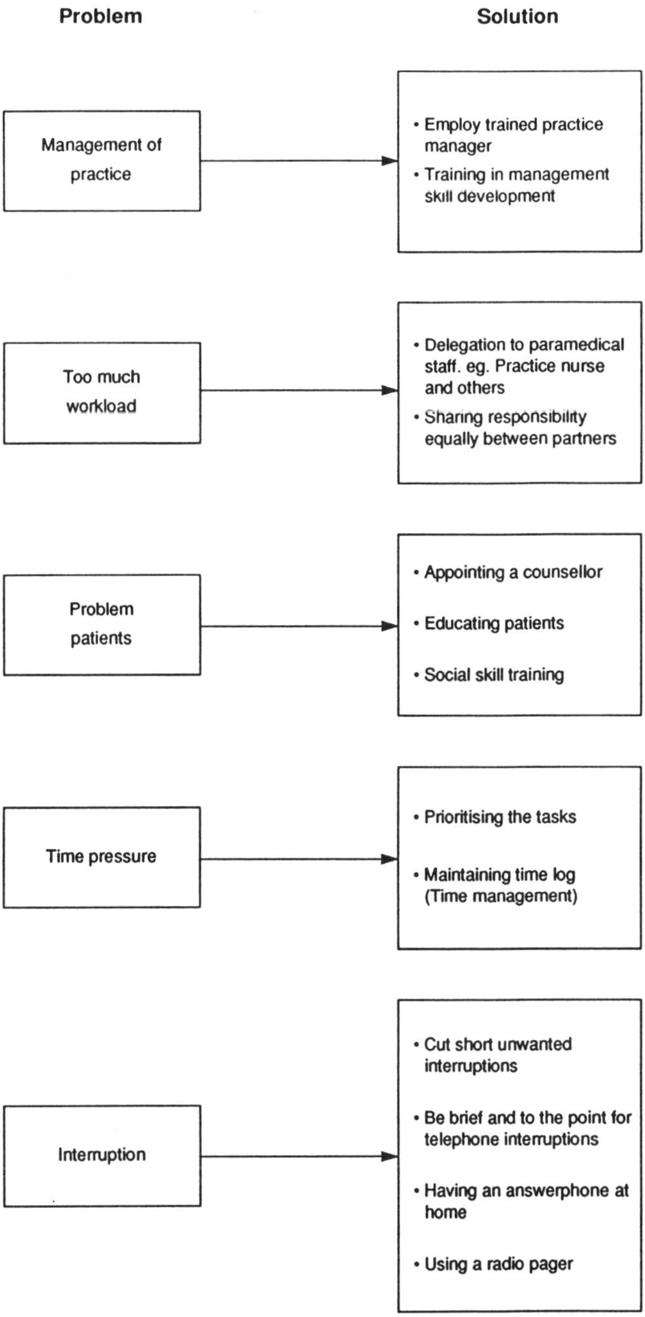

Figure 8.4. Coping with problems in general practice

Although only a small percentage of GPs were found to be alcoholic, the authors are concerned about this aspect, which may ultimately affect patient care. Such GPs can be encouraged to join Alcoholic Anonymous (AA), or other self-help groups and to take advantage of BMA counselling services.

Variations between GPs

Mental health and job satisfaction were found to be better for female GPs.

Female GPs are more satisfied with their job. Possibly they are part-time job holders and take less or no administrative responsibility than their male counterparts. Female GPs have much smaller lists, with an average of 1390 patients registered, compared with 2170 for male GPs [270]. Perhaps women GPs are better organised in order to cope with the combination of family, personal and practice commitments and responsibilities.

Male GPs were affected more by the factor 'demands of the job and patients expectations', while the female GPs were affected more by the factor 'home/work interface and social life'. Female GPs are possibly putting up with the conflict between work and home life at the expenses of their mental health. This could be due to their role as a woman/mother/wife resulting in additional responsibility at the domestic level. Flexibility in working hours is very important in order to fulfill domestic commitments. For a woman doctor it may be a stressful experience when returning to work after a career break for child-rearing. Provision should be made for retraining in order to re-gain confidence. As there are a growing number of women GPs in general practice their special needs should be recognised. Couples have to recognise each others professional commitment so that job sharing at home can be organised according to priorities and convenience.

It is worrying to find that male GPs showed a higher anxiety score than the UK normative sample. They should perhaps consider learning relaxation techniques and meditation in order to reduce their anxiety levels. This is discussed elsewhere in this chapter.

Overseas-qualified GPs showed more dissatisfaction in their job and more type A behaviour than their UK counterparts. This may reflect their medical training in their country of origin which may be predominantly clinical, with little social orientation. Anecdotal evidence suggests that most of them came to the UK with the intention of receiving specialist training in order to become specialists in the hospitals, but due to lack of opportunity may have entered into general practice instead. Due to their ethnic background, fear of discrimination, language difficulties, and lack of training in social skills they are perhaps compelled to work harder and faster in order to get parity with their UK-qualified colleagues. Special training designed for overseas-qualified GPs could be provided to increase their social skills.

GPs practising in urban areas were found to be more depressed, more dissatisfied in their job and had poorer mental health than the GPs practising in rural areas. It has already been mentioned that psychosocial problems are more prevalent in urban areas; also people move more frequently in urban areas and this can increase the GPs workload. Horobin and McIntosh [271] have found that shortage of time was a problem for 'urban' doctors but not for 'rural' doctors. Special incentives could be given to the GPs in urban areas to make their job attractive. As a positive step towards doctors working in deprived areas the government is now making a deprivation payment. In addition to our general recommendations (i.e. appointing a practice manager, a practice nurse, a counsellor and adequate staff) we suggest GPs may find it advantageous to learn time management skills as well.

Assaults on GPs during night visits are causing concern in several cities. GPs may consider calling for a police escort in suspected cases to avoid such episodes. A doctor's bag is an attraction for drug addicts. The GP could avoid carrying his case during night visits and instead use an unobtrusive bag with the minimum medicine. Finally additional allowances by the FHSAs should be considered for GPs in urban areas to enable them to take measures to protect their premises against vandalism.

What can the profession do?

To alleviate the effects of stress the profession has to acknowledge that there is a problem in the first place. At the level of the individual it can be suggested that GPs may try to adopt self-help methods (i.e. mental relaxation training, meditation, etc.) to cope with stress. According to Carruthers [151] "doctors must realise that the first people they must treat are themselves. This should increase their effectiveness".

Several courses on coping with stress aimed at the general public are offered throughout the country. These are based on a problem-solving approach to stress management and cover methods of diagnosis, skills training and action planning. Several of the methods focus upon dealing with the symptoms of stress and employ a variety of methods and approaches, often borrowed from behaviour therapy. GPs may find these courses useful in self-diagnosis of causes of stress and strengthening their areas of weakness.

Huntington [272] suggests a few management techniques to cut stress which might be helpful to GPs. She stressed the importance of the work environment and that the doctor must organise his workload that he has to deal with from day to day. The working environment could be kept pleasant through communication, collaboration and appropriate delegation.

At the organizational level a problem solving approach can be successfully implemented to reduce stress levels. In the first stage the areas of stress in the working environment has to be recognised by those representing the profession, by those in health service management and government so that subsequent intervention can be planned and directed as effectively as possible. In our study a number of such areas in the working environment have been identified. Therefore in the second stage planned intervention can be applied. In the light of our findings we shall elaborate three main areas: training; resources; and support.

Training

As stated earlier the results of our study suggest that the mental health and job satisfaction of GPs are affected by 'demands on the job and patients' expectations', 'interruptions', 'work/home conflict and social life', and 'administrative' responsibilities of the practice. All of these factors involve social and managerial skills, which can be developed by training. GPs can be trained in 'time management', 'people management', and 'organisational skills' development, as this might well help to overcome some of their job related stress. These skills should also assist them to minimise the impact of their job on their domestic life by allowing them more quality time at home. The social skills (to cope with patients), and the management skills (to administer their practice and deal with the increasing demands of their job) are already available from those used by industry [125] and could be easily adapted to help GPs cope better.

The GPs in this study frequently adopted negative coping strategies to cope with the pressures of work and home life which are counterproductive to their own health and society as a result. Adequate training should perhaps be provided to those wishing to enter into general practice during their medical training years and be continued during their general practice career as well so that they can cope better with the stresses of general practice.

Risks and failures are inevitable in the medical profession and training should be provided in the techniques of coping with blame when there is a failure. Stress management should be a part of the curriculum in undergraduate courses. Training should be provided to improve communication skills in doctors and to help them to break bad news to patients and their relatives.

As increasing numbers of medical students have chosen a career in general practice, more special departments should be created in medical schools, and those existing ones should be expanded in order to provide comprehensive training relevant to general practice. The introduction of mandatory vocational training in 1982 was a considerable step forward. But carefully designed evaluations of vocational training are essential to its impact on future practice. Emphasis should be given for continuing education in general practice so that the GPs can keep themselves up-to-date with recent medical advancements. The profession's leaders can help by persuading the Government to commit resources in order to provide proper continuing post-graduate education.

In the new GP contract the government has provided an allowance for post-graduate education to those GPs who attend a minimum number of hours of accredited courses. GPs have to attend these sessions to obtain their allowance but it is questionable whether their attendance is on their own initiative for education or just to sign the register to qualify for the allowance. As one GP in our interviews said "you can't compel people by a system of collecting points to educate themselves. There is a difference between educating yourself because you want to learn and just collecting points because you want the cash"!

Many of the doctors interviewed by us expressed their dissatisfaction that they were never taught the financial, managerial, and personnel skills which they felt were integral parts of the profession of general practice. GPs have to be managers as well as clinicians. If they are to take on managerial roles they have to be clear about the financial status of the practice such as surgery expenses, ancillary staff costs and how these are to be recouped. There are several professional organisations offering their services to GPs. Those who have never had any training in management can now use these organisations to get professional advice.

The work in general practice is unique. The anxiety created by the degree of urgency of many decisions, and the uncertain environment in which the work takes place require a high level of management skills to keep services running. In order to achieve long term objectives a high degree of ability is required to prioritise the task and not to be distracted by crises. Good planning and management skills are necessary for general practice. There are certain management functions in which the GP must take part, such as determining policies, planning, and decision making. Again training in delegation and other management skills should be provided during the training period.

The other area where the GP faces difficulty is with problem solving skills, such as psycho-social problems, and relationship problems. These are areas where specific training may be devoted during vocational training.

Resources

The result of our study showed that GPs are not satisfied with their rate of pay. This may be due to their financial commitments and lack of resources to improve the surgery premises and update with modern equipment in order to improve patient care. Under the present terms of their contract GPs may not be allowed to reimburse their expenses if they employ an electrocardiogram (ECG) technician and/or counsellors to ease their burden although some FHSAs do allow reimbursement for counsellors. The GPs' time and knowledge could well be spent on patient care instead of dealing with non-medical psychological problems that could be dealt with by a counsellor. This makes sense financially, as a counsellor can be employed at much less expense than a doctor. However, a recent study by Sibbald *et al.* [273] found that although counselling services in general practice are widespread the counsellors lacked qualifications. They comment that although counsellors may have acquired the skill to deal with a certain range of problems it is unlikely that any one counsellor will have the qualifications to deal with the wide range of problems seen in general practice.

Anecdotal evidence suggests that the most feared item in the contract is fund holding. It is worth noting a comment by a GP:

> "We are very concerned that there have been no pilot studies done on what effect of budget holding is going to be. Without trials we just don't know what the effect will be." [274]

It is feared that fund holding will usher in a 'new age of medicine' in which GPs will think more in financial terms than about the welfare of the patients. Another GP comments:

> "This thing has simply not been thought through enough. It will take us back to the old pool system of robbing Peter to pay Paul, one doctor living off another." [274]

The new contract promises more involvement from FHSAs in deciding which ancillary staff they employ in their practices. GPs are very worried about this fearing that cash-limited FHSAs will be forced to interfere more and more in the running of general practice in order to protect their budgets. Here is a GP's comment:

> "The FHSAs will have to use their powers because they will have to account to central government for every penny they spend. They are going to be hamstrung. They have a budget and they will have to stick to it." [275]

He also voiced that "the FPCs will be forced to use powers to exert more control on GPs, and general practice will be similar to running a 'franchise restaurant'". The result in our pre-contract study showed that the greatest source of satisfaction for GPs was associated with the freedom to choose working methods. It seems to us that the job satisfaction on freedom of choice is being reduced.

The proportion of NHS gross expenditure spent on general medical services fell from 10.1% in 1949 to 7.1% in 1983 [276]. Financial allocations for spending in acute hospital services should not be reduced further. As primary care teams are made to take more responsibility resources should be provided to meet the demand. To achieve its aims the government should provide adequate resources for the NHS as a whole and allocate a greater proportion to general practice.

Financial reward to individuals is recognised as important in most avenues of life and good performance is usually rewarded by better pay in most occupations. The government must take the responsibility to provide the resources necessary for better terms of service and financial rewards for GPs.

Support

Incapacity to cope with stress and the inability to seek help should not be considered as a weakness but a strength; recognition of stress is the first step forward in stress management. Doctors are often reluctant and uncooperative patients and are also likely to deny depression and psychological illness [239]. Doctors should leave the stigma behind and come forward for help.

The National Counselling Service for Sick Doctors has handled 450 calls since its inception in 1985 [277]. Its services are open to all medical practitioners in the UK and calls are accepted from sick doctors, worried colleagues and spouses. It is funded by the Government and managed by a small independent committee of management which provides a humane and constructive approach to the sick doctor whose competence to practice has been eroded. In general practice, the FHSAs and LMCs (Local Medical Committees) may intervene when concern has been raised about a local colleague. Relatively small numbers of cases are dealt with by these statutory arrangements compared with the numbers handled by the counselling service [277].

National advisors are drawn from all branches of medicine and include 60 GPs nominated by the RCGP and GMSC and are distributed throughout the UK. When a call is received the only detail taken at the centre is the area in which the GP works. The name and phone number of one or more GP advisors is given to the referrer who is encouraged to contact the advisor and discuss the problem. Advisors need to be aware of any arrangements taken locally to meet the problem. If the sick doctor is willing to accept help, the national advisor may undertake the task or call upon one of 250 counsellors working for the service to become involved.

The General Medical Council has been operating a scheme to help doctors who are impaired by reason of mental or physical illness. It may consider retaining the doctor on the Medical Register dependent upon the doctor receiving medical attention. The Council has approved a two year experimental scheme under which liaison advisers are available to give additional advice and assistance to those doctors who are under the council's health procedures.

The National Association for Staff Support (NASS) is a registered charity consisting of professionals coordinating and developing staff support resources for all health care staff. The Association has produced a number of reports on stress management within the health services and has contacts all over the country who can provide help and advice on staff support services.

In America, a growing number of medical schools and residency programmes are providing courses for medical students to understand the pressures of the inherent susceptibility in medical practice before any serious problems develop. The American Academy of Family Physicians (AAFP) has programmes to deal with physician's stress. The Committee has focused on the effect of stress on residents and practising physicians. Other organisations also have similar programmes for practising physicians. It can be suggested that British medical schools should provide courses for their students to understand the inherent stress of medicine and introduce different coping skills to reduce pressure.

Attempts have been made in the UK to provide support service for physicians suffering from stress at work [236]. The 'three wise men', is a Committee which investigates complaints within the profession about doctors who exhibit difficulties in their functioning, such as drinking problems and drug addiction. This system has, however, tended to penalise and reprimand physicians rather than providing some form of coping support [236]. The General Medical Council is actively involved to provide some service to rehabilitate them. But without an establishment of a definite and formal social support system stress-related psychological and physical problems may continue among doctors. GPs need to receive positive support from their senior colleagues but since seeking help may be interpreted as admission of inadequacy, which may affect their career, there should be provision for external counselling.

We suggest that practices can introduce a 'support network' system for problem solving. A group practice of eight doctors could form four colleague pairs, so that when a problem is experienced by one of them he can feel free to discuss it with a fellow colleague in a non-threatening and comfortable way, but if no solution is found then this pair may wish to involve one of the other pairs. Ultimately the whole group may meet and try to solve the problem. If all fails then outside help may be required. There should be a local support group of GPs who can share each others problem comfortably. Practices should also have a policy on partners' problems and ill health. Informal time should be made available for the parties to get to know each other socially. Everyone should be encouraged to express their feelings. They should never deny or repress a problem.

The family is a major source of support for the GP, providing the problem solving, listening and accepting behaviours that are essential to alleviate stresses, even though they may be unable to change the circumstances that created them. Myers, Lindethal and Pepper [278] found that people who were more integrated in society (i.e. being married with children and of higher socio-economic status) coped better with different negative life crises than those not as integrated. Therefore, it is necessary for the GP's family (especially spouse) to try to understand his problems in order to overcome the factors contributing to stress. Also the GP must learn to share himself as a person with the family.

Changing type A behaviour

The results of this study clearly indicate that there is an obvious need for the introduction of type A behaviour modification programmes for GPs. Type A behaviour modification programmes with both CHD patients and healthy individuals have shown significant reduction in serum cholesterol levels and blood pressure, lower frequencies of subsequent CHD, increased work productivity and improved family relationships [279,280,282].

GPs who suffer from 'hurry sickness' or chronic type A behaviour, may find the following suggestions as helpful coping strategies. Friedman and Rosenman [148] recommend a number of 'drills against hurry sickness', which they claim work for their type A patients. We now consider some suggestions from their unique book 'Type A Behaviour and Your Heart'.

1. *Force yourself to listen to others*. Drill: 'Begin in your vocational hours to listen quietly to the conversation of other people. Quit trying to finish their sentences. An even better sort of drill for you if you have been in the habit of hastening the other person's speech rhythm is to seek out a person who stutters and then deliberately remain tranquil.'

2. *Think before saying something*. Drill: '(a) Do I really have anything important to say? (b) Does anyone want to hear it? (c) Is this the time to say it? If the answer to any of these three questions is 'no', then remain quiet even if you find yourself biting your lips in frustration.'

3. *Change your obsessional time directed behaviour.* Drill: 'Whenever you catch yourself speeding up your car in order to get through a yellow light at an intersection, penalize yourself by immediately turning right at the next corner. Circle the block and approach the same corner and signal right again. After such penalization you may find yourself racing a yellow light a second, but probably not a third time.' Drill: 'Purposely, with a companion, frequent restaurants and theatres where you know there will be a period of waiting. If your companion happens to be your partner, remember that you spend far longer periods of time alone with him/her in your own home without fidgeting. If you and your companion cannot find enough to say to each other as you sit and wait in a restaurant or theatre, then you had both better seek different companions.'

4. *Carry out exercises to assess your type A behaviour.* Drill: 'Perhaps one of the most important new habits you can establish is to review at least once a week the original causes of your present 'hurry sickness'.' In other words, try to get to the source of your problems and current obsessions, to the reasons for your time-dominated behaviour. Is it a need to feel important? Is it designed to avoid some activity or person? Is it really essential to the success of a particular personal or organizational goal? In respect to this latter point, never forget when confronted by any task to ask yourself the following questions: (a) Will this matter have importance five years from now? (b) Must I do this right now, or do I have enough time to think about the best way to accomplish it?'

5. *Slow down yourself.* Drill: 'Tell yourself at least once a day that no enterprise ever failed because it was executed too slowly, too well. Ask yourself, are good judgement and correct decisions best formulated under unhurried circumstances or under deadline pressures?'

6. *Widen your outside activities.* Drill: 'Attempt to read books that demand not only your entire attention but also a certain amount of patience. We have repeatedly advised our type A patients to attempt reading Proust's seven volume novel *The Rememberance of Times Past* not because it is one of the great modern classics (which it is), but because the author needs several chapters to describe an event that most type A subjects would have handled in a sentence or two.'

7. Avoid making unnecessary appointments and protect your time – learn to say 'no'. 'Try to never forget that if you fail to protect your allotment of time no one else will. And the older you become the more important the truth is.'

8. *Stress-free breathing spaces.* Drill: Take as many stress-free 'breathing spaces' during the course of an intensive working day as is possible. 'Learn to interrupt long or even short sessions of any type of activity that you know or suspect may induce tension and stress before it is finished. Such stress is particularly apt to arise in the course of writing long memos, reports or articles.'

9. *Appreciate others.* Drill: 'Begin to speak your thanks or appreciation to others when they have performed services for you. And do not do so, like so many hostile type A subjects, with merely a grunt of thanks.'

In summary, the above suggestions involve such exercises as relaxation and behavioural speed changes. Additional specific behavioural drills can be introduced at the work place e.g. having fewer meetings, scheduling telephone calls, allotting free-time periods, and so on [148,281,282]. It would appear that GPs who have the behavioural characteristics of type A have a somewhat higher likelihood of being over stressed. However, GPs who have this type A behaviour pattern appear to be able to avoid the feelings of being over-stressed if they can adopt some kind of relaxation practice.

Suinn [282] conducted a behaviour modification programme for those who were Type A and had cardiac problems and were distinctly under stress. They were put through an experimental-based cardiac stress management training programme designed to change their type A behavioural pattern which consisted of a variety of relaxation exercises discussed later in this chapter thereby re-educating the individual to control his environment. After the programme it was shown that most type As had more control over their stress, had lower blood pressure levels and they seemed to develop a style of living which was less hurried and more controlled.

Relaxation methods

GPs can learn techniques that help them to relax. This is an important skill to acquire and deploy in counteracting the physical reactions to stress such as increased heart rate, raised blood pressure and higher muscle tension. Transcendental meditation (TM) has been acknowledged to be a highly efficient stress reducing technique. TM reduces stress, and the reduction in stress levels helps to increase productivity and efficiency at work. Individuals who operate at relatively low levels of stress appear to enjoy their work, to get on well with other individuals and to be more effective at their jobs.

After several years of investigating TM and the impact of TM upon stress reduction, Benson [283] began a serious attempt to develop another technique, named secular meditation, which duplicated the results of TM. Benson's approach utilises four elements which are almost universal within meditation techniques.

1. Choose a calm, quiet environment
2. Sit in a comfortable position in a comfortable chair
3. Assume a passive attitude
4. Meditate (on an object on which to focus mentally)

The meditation technique suggested by Benson utilises a single and universal mantra (the sacred word), the word 'one'. Meditators are told to breathe in through the nose, and then to breathe out while silently repeating the word 'one'. Benson suggests that his technique be continued for approximately 20 minutes and practised once or twice a day but not within two hours of a meal. His research findings indicate that the technique shares many of the same benefits of TM. Benson [283] recommended that the relaxation response 'can act as a built-in method of counteracting the stresses of everyday living which bring forth the fight-or-flight response'.

Other techniques involve making the individual aware of his body's reaction to stress, whether it be physiological or psychological. Two techniques have been recognised to help individuals with stressful behaviour to reduce their stress – through 'anxiety management training' and 'viscio-motor behaviour rehearsal'. The individual is made aware of the onset of anxiety usually indicated by tightening of the muscles or increase in heart rate and he is then taught to reduce this stress through training in muscle relaxation. Suinn [282] found this method to be effective in lowering stress in individuals faced with a variety of different personal and occupational problems.

Another technique is biofeedback, in which the body's internal responses are made externally visible. Biofeedback training uses instruments to help the individual control responses of the autonomic nervous system. For example, the individual monitors an auditory signal of his own heart rate and experiments with different thoughts and feelings to slow the heart rate. Once he learns to recognise the feelings associated with the reduction of the heart rate then the instrument is removed and the individual tries to control the heart rate without it. Perhaps one of the most powerful, but least understood methods of stress reduction is the practice of yoga. Like TM, yoga evokes illusions of Indian culture. And like TM, the practising of yoga is actually a very simple, clear cut mechanism which is not really bound to a particular culture or religion. In fact the efficient practice of yoga requires both a disciplined mind and body.

While relaxation is a generally useful skill and can help interrupt stress effects, a similar effect can be achieved more readily by physical release processes such as stretching, yawning and shaking [284]. The addition of positive focussing to these or any form of relaxation will increase the effects. The use of cathartic discharge, achieved by humour, which disrupts the negative thinking components of stress is another technique which is more time effective than teaching relaxation alone [284].

Individuals are able to deal with stress if they are physically fit. Therefore, it can be recommended for GPs to do a little light exercise every other day. There is no need to push themselves too hard, the aim is to avoid being too sedentary. By adopting a healthy lifestyle with regular meals of healthy food and restricting alcoholic drinks they will help to minimise stress.

A stress diary

Establishing the sources of stress and strain is not always easy. It is important for GPs to be able to identify precisely those individual or series of related events that may be causing stress or tension. One way of doing this is to maintain a stress diary for a few weeks, noting all activities and using a simple code to indicate the strain involved. This should provide information about the type of incident or person or situation that causes the individual most difficulty. An awareness of this should help the GP to develop an action plan to minimise or eliminate the stressors (see Table 8.1).

Table 8.1. Sample stress diary

Date	Time	Type of incident	People involved	Type of situation	What you did	What you should have done
Week 1						
Monday						
Tuesday						
Wednesday						
Thursday						
Friday						
Saturday						
Sunday						

For example, at the end of a few weeks review the incidents and people involved which caused the most stress and try to isolate particular events and specific people who consistently seem to be implicated in stressful work experiences; systematically think through the options or alternative methods of coping.

Time management

According to Jack Ferner [286] time management is "efficient use of our resources, including time, in such a way that we are effective in achieving important personal goals". Several surveys have looked into GPs utilization of time, revealing 'wide variety' as a common factor. There may be no direct relationship between a doctor's list size and work pattern and quality of health care provided. A doctor with a large list size may be efficient and satisfy his patients' needs whereas a doctor with a small list size may have to work hard and become a slave to demands. Implementing good time management will not only benefit the GP but his patients as well.

The following steps are recommended for GPs to practice time management in general.

1. Identify key areas where you need to spend most of your time.

2. Work out an acceptable balance of work and relaxation.

3. Try to have sometime for each day that is for you.

4. Plan your time, prioritise your tasks and try to build some flexibility (class 1 activities are the highest priority (must do); class 2 are 'should do' areas; and class 3 are 'might do' areas which can wait).

5. Set yourself realistic achievable goals.

6. Keep your regular work sessions short. Several short sessions usually achieve more than one long session.

7. If you have difficulty getting started then examine what you are doing to cause delay, e.g. tidying desk, having a cup of coffee, having another cup of coffee, seeing drug representative, going through morning mail.

8. Handle each piece of paper only once and scan journals quickly.

9. Try taking short breaks (10 minutes) half-way through surgeries.

10. Perfection eats up time. Learn to be satisfied with the best you can do in the time available.

11. Be kind to yourself – do not demand too much of yourself if you are not well or under stress.

12. Keep and analyse a time log for four weeks in which you record how you actually spend your time and whether this is how you wish to spend it.

An example of time log for GPs

Time		**Surgery activity**	**Other activities (specify)**
Start	**Finish**		

Finally, there are numerous books and seminars which give useful tips for dealing with time-management problems.

Time management for meetings

In order to cope with the frequent changes in the NHS, the new GP contract, and fund holding GPs are having to spend much more of their time in meetings. Some may be unnecessary and others could be carried out in a rapid, informal way allowing discussion and information-sharing without wasting time. Therefore the most important step is to avoid attending any meeting which is not absolutely necessary, and only hold a meeting if there is something definite to discuss.

Ways to save time at meetings:

Attend those meetings which are absolutely necessary.
Be punctual and don't wait for latecomers.
Consider only attending the relevant part of the meeting.
Decide which partners will follow-up individual points.
Emphasise avoiding interruptions unless they are urgent
Finishing and starting time to be fixed for each meeting.
Give consideration as to whether a letter, fax or phone call would achieve the same goal as a meeting.
Have a look at the agenda before meetings to prepare yourself.
Insist on taking minutes as you go along.
Just don't make a habit of attending meetings.

Some simple stress management techniques

To avoid stress:

- Accept it is normal to be an imperfect person in an imperfect world.

- The adaptive approach is to separate thoughts from feelings and put situations in perspective. Problems are analysed logically and plans made to resolve them.

- Work out those situations and people which cause you stress and why.

- Change those things that actually can be changed.

- Identify and respect your own good points.

- Improve your shortcomings as much as possible and then accept them as part of you.

- Don't compare yourself with others.

- Set realistic goals – tackle big problems one step at a time, expect to make mistakes, apologise and then learn from them.

- One may delegate tasks but one cannot delegate responsibility.

- Look at ways to delegate jobs that are urgent but not important, but if you delegate important activities, follow them up to ensure they are done correctly.

- Running late in surgeries may be helped by starting on time, revising appointment time and also avoiding interruptions.

- Assertiveness training is particularly helpful for people who have difficulty in saying 'no'.

Coping with the new contract

During the period June to September 1992 we conducted in-depth interviews on a sample of 49 GPs in the North-West of England to try and find out the major sources and levels of stress. The sample contained 36 male and 13 female GPs and the details of the study are given in Appendix 22. Although the GPs were selected randomly from each FHSA list, the areas were chosen non-randomly and this may restrict the general applicability of the data. We believe, however, that the results reflect the views of many GPs within the north-west region.

The GPs were asked to identify potential causes of stress, both at work, at home and socially (as suggested by Cooper and Marshall [58]. In addition to the previous stressors mentioned in Chapter 5, the following are new stressors found after the introduction of the new contract.

1. Increased paperwork
2. Lack of consultation over reforms
3. New phenomenon of business stress being experienced by GPs
4. Imposition of indicative prescribing
5. Extra contractual referrals
6. An increased emphasis on screening, administration and accounting
7. Increased litigation
8. Fund holding management
9. Patients charter
10. Increased performance, expectations from FHSA and peers
11. Threat of financial clawback
12. On-going audit

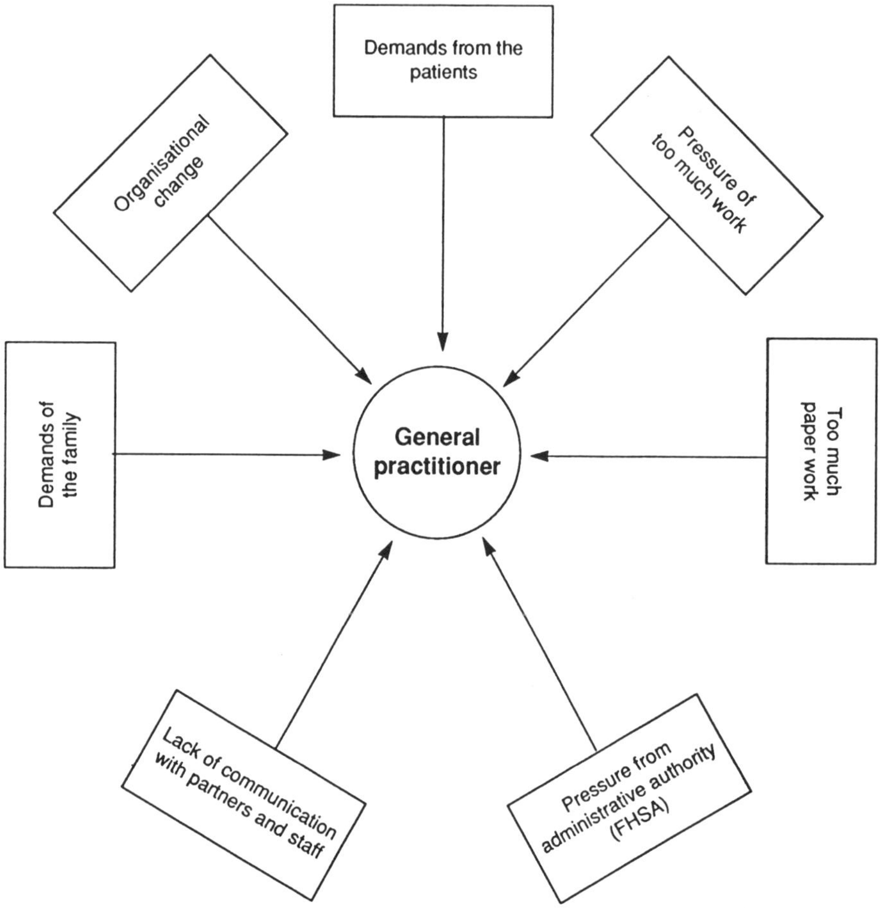

Figure 8.5. Stressors affecting the GP at work after the introduction of the new contract

We have briefly mentioned some of the changes in the new GP contract and their implications in the first chapter. Here, we put forward our views and comments, and some suggestions gathered from GPs during post contract interviews, regarding adaptation to the new contract. These are merely general views which may not be applicable to all practices but GPs may find them helpful in organising their practices to meet the demands of the new contract. Figure 8.5 shows the major stressors affecting the GP at work after the introduction of the new contract. Some specific suggestions are as follows:

Immunization

Pregnant mothers may be motivated during the antenatal period to bring their babies for immunization to the surgery instead of taking the babies to the local Health Authority clinics. They should also be encouraged to give their option to the health visitor that they wish their babies to be immunized in their own GP surgeries. Doctors or practice managers may find it a good idea to send congratulations cards to the mothers with a note reminding them to bring their babies to the immunization clinic on a particular day. Uptake can be increased by giving parents a realistic appraisal of risks and benefits of vaccination and offering advice on preparing a child for the immunisation.

Cervical cytology

Some practices may have made their policies on cervical cytology prior to the implementation of the new contract and may have achieved their targets without much difficulty. But other practices have expressed their dissatisfaction for having not been able to achieve their targets. It is important to match the practice list with that of the FHSA and ensure that 'ghost' patients who may otherwise affect the target percentage have been removed. A list of hysterectomised women should also be maintained who are then excluded from the target population. A computerised or well-organised manual recall register for cervical smear would help the practice to contact women due for their smears. Some practices resmear their patients every three years although government advice is for this to be done every five years for payment purposes. Recall requests may be sent up to three times and defaulters may be approached by the practice nurse personally to talk to the patients, answer any queries and deal with any fears they may have.

Postgraduate education allowance (PGEA)

There is tremendous pressure on GPs to complete ten PGEA sessions in a year (30 hours according to the modified rule) to be fully eligible for PGEA so that they can be compensated for the financial loss due to the cut in seniority payments. We feel that as an alternative GPs may wish to attend courses to complete the full ten sessions in one go, either inside the UK or abroad, which are organised at holiday centres. Families would then be able to go together and may not feel quite so neglected.

Night visits

It is well known that disrupted sleep leads to tiredness and causes impairment of judgement the following day. Although the higher rate of payments for night visits may tempt some GPs to do their own calls it may damage their health and impair their ability to conduct their surgeries satisfactorily. Alternatively using a deputising service to cover night calls can be expensive. As a compromise one may choose to take the night calls up to a certain time (e.g. around midnight) and then pass on the calls to the deputising services. This would enable a complete rest until the next morning. It could also be suggested that in some areas specially designed 'emergency centres' staffed by GPs may be set up, within convenient reach of the practice area, to provide out-of-hours primary medical care. Patients requiring medical attention would be advised to attend such centres but provision still has to be made to visit those patients at their own place if they are housebound or unable to travel.

Health promotion clinics

Agreements may be reached with the FHSA for health promotion clinics to be conducted by the practice nurse under the supervision of the GP. It is then possible in a group practice that only one GP needs to be present in the practice premises to be available to the practice nurse to give advice if needed. In this way several health promotion clinics can be conducted to provide better health care cover. Health promotion clinics such as keep-fit, relaxation, swimming etc. can serve both the purposes of being classified as a clinic and benefiting patients' health and quality of life, and also give a chance to GPs and staff for exercise and relaxation as well.

Annual reports

GPs are required to produce annual reports to the FHSA with the detailed information on their individual staff and other aspects of the practice. These details can either be processed by the practice computer or be completed manually. Statistical packages are now available to record the above information with minimal effort. The completed sheets can then be passed onto the practice manager who can compile the data at the end of the year to produce the annual report.

Computers in general practice

Use of computers is not compulsory but GPs have been encouraged to use this aspect of modern information technology through generous reimbursement schemes. It is, however, a basic requirement for fund holders. Some GPs have expressed their dissatisfaction at the lack of adequate technical support, diversion of attention during consultation and the initial financial outlay. It is advisable to choose a system which includes hardware, software and maintenace by a single company as it is often the case that when a problem occurs, the responsibility is shifted to others if multiple companies are involved. Reluctant colleagues could be motivated and encouraged to attend basic training courses.

Community care

"Over the past two years much anxiety has been generated within the profession that the transfer of community care would increase workload, threaten the doctor–patient relationship and reduce GP's to working for local authorities" [285]. The final decision has now been taken by the government and fund allocation has been announced. The profession is relieved that the social services department will be responsible for assessing the needs of an individual and arranging 'care packages'. GPs are obliged to provide basic factual information to the local authority and advice to patients about how they can avail themselves of services provided by their local social services department. Community care has been included in the budget of fund holding practices to be effective from April 1993. This is an additional workload for them but they can best deal with this by joint consultation with other fundholding practices or even better by forming a consortium.

Fund holding

Fund holding, despite opposition from the BMA, is growing in momentum. More and more GPs are being encouraged into fund holding, many of them agreeing less out of a commitment to its principle than from a fear of being left behind.

Initially only practices with at least 11,000 patients were considered for fundholding but the limit has now been relaxed and it is expected that this will be further reduced to include practices with 7000 patients in the third wave (April 1993).

The preparatory year for prospective fundholders is hectic due to numerous meetings and administrative work and this will be more so for the prospective third wave fund holders due to the inclusion of community care services from April 1993. Practices might consider nominating one of their partners as an 'executive partner' who would take the responsibility of monitoring progress during the preparatory year and keeping other partners informed. He could be given time off from the surgery whenever need arises so that he can keep the administrative work up-to-date.

The future

It is evident that general practice is likely to remain a high stress occupation and further changes in the NHS are likely to occur in the future. Increased stress levels following the introduction of the new contract may not solely be attributed to it but it can be assumed that its implementation at an accelerated rate with the loss of the professions control at the work place may have been one of the contributing factors. However, a sensible way to absorb the changes and adapt to it is to think positively. Major changes such as fund holding may be considered as a challenge and opportunity to control the working environment and develop skills to match with the demands. GPs mental health must remain sound if they are expected to provide comprehensive health care to their patients. Stress must be recognised in relation to the ability of the GP to tolerate it, the personality of the individual GP and the way he perceives and interacts with the environment. GPs who adapt a palliative coping strategy may feel the short term response as personally desirable and less costly than altering the demands. It may not however be possible to alter the demands as some of the factors are considered as inherent to the job such as 'interruptions' but it can be suggested that adaptation to the environment needs change within the individual and acquiring skills in dealing with it.

As Maslach says "we do not yet know the relative importance of each dimension to answer such questions as does the nature of the job have a greater importance than individuals personality or vice versa, nor do we know just how one dimension influences the other" [48].

It is desirable to conduct further studies by collecting both subjective and objective data in order to substantiate or refute the findings of our previous studies on stress among GPs. However, since our post-contract interview findings we have conducted a nationwide quantitative survey, the results of which are in the process of analysis.It remains to be seen if the dust has settled and GPs' stress levels have altered.

References

1. British Medical Association General Medical Services Committee. General Practice – A British Success. London, BMA. 1983.
2. Leeuwenhorst Working Party. The work of the general practitioner: statement by a working party of the 2nd European Conference on the teaching of general practice. J R Coll Gen Pract. 1977;27:117.
3. Central Health Services Council. General Practice within the National Health Service. Report of the Committee on General Practice (Chairman: Professor Sir Henry Cohen), London, HMSO. 1954.
4. Last JM, Stanley GR. Career preferences of young British doctors. Br J Med Educ. 1968;2:137–55.
5. Parkhouse J, McLaughlin C. Career preferences of doctors graduating in 1974. Br Med J. 1976;ii:630–32.
6. Parkhouse J, Howard M. A follow up of the career preferences of Manchester and Sheffield graduates of 1972 & 1973. J Med Educ. 1978;12:377–81.
7. Pulse. October 10, 1992.
8. British Medical Association. Primary health care teams, Board of Science and Education. 1974.
9. Cartwright A, Anderson R. 1981. General Practice Revisited. London: Tavistock.
10. Social Trends. London: HMSO. 1992.
11. Department of Health and Social Security. Health and personal social services statistics for England. London: HMSO, 1985.
12. Reedy BLEC. The health team. In Fry J, ed. Trends in General Practice. For the Royal College of General Practitioners by the British Medical Journal, London. 1977:111–36.
13. Hasler JC, Hemphill PMR, Stewart TI, Boyle N, Harris A, Palmer E. Development of the nursing section of the community health team. Br Med J. 1968;iii:734–6.
14. Fry J, Brooks D, McColl I. NHS Data Book. Lancaster: MTP Press. 1984.
15. Health Department of Great Britain. General Practice in the NHS. The 1990 Contract. August 1989.
16. Pulse. April 6, 1991.
17. Financial Pulse. June 2, 1991.
18. GP. April 5, 1991.
19. Pirie A, Kelly M. Fund holding: a practice guide 1992. Radcliffe Medical Press, p.1.
20. General Practitioner. September 18, 1992.
21. Hinkle LE. The concept of 'stress' in the biological and social sciences. Sci Med Man. 1973;1:31–48.
22. Cannon WG. Bodily Changes in Pain, Hunger, Fear and Rage: An Account of Recent Researches into the Function of Emotional Excitement, 2nd edn. New York: Appleton. 1929.
23. Appley MH, Trumbull R. On the concept of psychological stress. In Appley MH, Trumbull R (ed). Psychological Stress. New York: Meredith Publishing Company. 1967.
24. Selye H. The evolution of the stress concept. Am Sci. 1973;61:692–9.
25. Selye H. Stress Without Distress. New York: Lippincott. 1974.
26. Selye H. Stress in Health and Disease. London: Butterworths. 1976.
27. Lazarus R. The concept of stress and disease. In Levi L, ed. Society, Stress and Disease. London: Oxford University Press. 1971:53–60.
28. Selye H. A syndrome produced diverse nocuous agents. Nature. 1936;138:32.
29. Selye H. The Stress of Life. USA: McGraw-Hill. 1956.
30. Selye H. The stress concept: past, present and future. In Cooper CL, ed. Stress Research: Issues for the eighties. London: John Wiley & Sons. 1980.
31. Mechanic D. Practice orientations among general medical practitioners in England and Wales. Med Care. 1970;8:15–25.
32. Cox T. Stress. London: McMillan. 1978.
33. Selye H. Stress. Montreal, Acta. 1950.
34. Lacey JI. Somatic response patterning and stress: some revisions of activation theory. In Appley MH, Trumbull R, eds. Psychological Stress. New York: Appleton-Century-Crofts. 1967.
35. Mason JW. A reevaluation of the concept of 'non-specificity' in stress theory. J Psychiatr Res. 1971;8:323–3.
36. McGrath JE. A conceptual formulation for research on stress. In McGrath JE, ed. Social and Psychological Factors on Stress. New York: Rinehart and Winston. 1970:10–21.
37. Holmes TH, Rahe RH. The social readjustment rating scale. J Psychosom Res. 1967;11:213–8.

38. Lazarus R. Patterns of Adjustment. New York: McGraw-Hill. 1976.
39. Lazarus RS. Psychological Stress and the Coping Process. New York: McGraw-Hill. 1966.
40. Van Harrison R. Job stress as person environment misfit. A symposium presented at the 84th Annual Convention of the American Psychological Association, Michigan. 1976.
41. Cooper CL. The Stress Check. Englewood Cliffs, New Jersey: Prentice-Hall. 1981.
42. French JRP. Person-role fit. In Maclean A, ed. Occupational Stress. Springfield, Illinois: Charles C Thomas. 1974.
43. French JRP, Rogers W, Cobb S. A model of person environment fit. In Coelho GW, Hamburgh DA, Adams JE, eds. Coping and Adaption. New York: Basic Books. 1974.
44. French JR, Caplan RD, Van Harrison R. The Mechanisms of Job Stress and Strain. John Wiley & Sons. 1982.
45. Hingley P, Cooper CL. Stress and the Nurse Manager. Chichester: John Wiley & Sons. 1986.
46. Cooper CL, Marshall J. Sources of managerial and white collar stress. In Cooper CL, Payne R, eds. Stress at Work. Chichester: John Wiley & Sons. 1978:81–105.
47. Pulse. January 23, 1988.
48. Maslach C, Jackson SE. Burnout in health professions: A social psychological analysis. In: Sanders GS, Suls J, eds., Social psychology of health and illness. Erlbaum: Hillsdale, NJ. pp. 227–54.
49. Lazarus R, Folkman S. Stress, Appraisal and Coping. New York: Springer-Verlag. 1984.
50. Folkman S, Lazarus RS. An analysis of coping in a middle-aged community sample. J Health Soc Behav. 1980;21:219–39.
51. Kelly D. Professional burnout. Update. 1992;44(12):1163–70.
52. Lazarus R. The costs and benefits of denial. In Breznitz S, ed. The Denial of Stress. New York: International Universities Press. 1983.
53. Lazarus R. The trivialisation of distress. In Rosen JC, Solomon LJ, eds. Preventing Health Risk Behaviours and Promoting Coping with Illness. 1983:8.
54. House JS. Work Stress and Social Support. USA: Addison-Wesley. 1981.
55. Lazarus R. The stress and coping paradigm. In Eisdorfer C, Cohen D, Kleinman A, Maxim P, eds. Models for Clinical Psychopathology. New York: Spectrum. 1981.
56. Cooper CL, Cooper RF, Faragher EB. A prospective study of the relationship between breast cancer and life events, Type A behaviour, social support and coping skills. Stress Med. 1986;2:271–7.
57. Flanagan CM. People and change: an introduction to counselling and stress management. Lawrence Erlbaum Associates. 1990.
58. Cooper CL, Marshall J. Occupational sources of stress. A review of the literature relating to coronary heart disease and mental ill health. J Occup Psychol. 1976;49:11–28.
59. Porter AMD, Howie JGR, Levinson AS. Stress and the general practitioner. In Payne R, Firth-Cozens J, eds. Stress in Health Professionals. Chichester: Wiley. 1987:45–70.
60. Rout U. Occupational Stress in General Practice. MSc Dissertation, UMIST. 1986.
61. Rout U. Occupational Stress in General Practitioner. PhD Thesis, UMIST. 1989.
62. Cooper CL, Rout U, Faragher B. Mental health, job satisfaction and job stress among general practitioners. Br Med J. 1989;293:366–70.
63. Makin PJ, Rout U, Cooper CL. Job satisfaction and occupational stress in general practitioners: A pilot study. J R Coll Gen Pract. 1988;38:303–6.
64. Sutherland VJ, Cooper CL. Job stress, satisfaction and mental health among GPs before and after introduction of new contract. Br Med J. 1992;304:1545–8.
65. Morris JN, Heady JA, Barley RG. Coronary heart disease in medical practitioners. Br Med J. 1952;1:503–20.
66. Allibone A, Oakes D, Shannon HS. The health and health care of doctors. J R Coll Gen Pract. 1981;31:728–34.
67. McCue JD. The effects of stress on physicians and their medical practice. N Engl J Med. 1982;458–63.
68. Linn LS, Yager J, Cope D, Leake B. Health status, job satisfaction, job stress and life satisfaction among academic and clinical faculty. JAMA. 1985;254:2775–82.
69. Krakowski AJ. Stress and the practice of medicine: II, Stressors, stresses and strains. Psychother Psychosom. 1982;38:11–23.
70. Crammond WA. Aust NZ Med J. 1969;3:324. Cited in Murray R. J R Coll Physicians. 1978;12(5).
71. Glaser BG, Strauss AL. Awareness of Dying. 1966. London: Weidenfeld and Nicholson.
72. Cartwright A, Hockey L, Anderson JL. Life before death. London: Routledge and Kegan Paul. 1973.
73. Cartwright A. Patients and their doctor. Routledge & Kegan Paul: London, 1977.
74. Rankin HJ, Serieys NM, Elliot-Binns CP. Determinants of mood in general practitioners. Br Med J.

1987;295:618–20.
75. Harris AC. Violence in general practice. Br Med J. 1989;298:63–4.
76. D'Ursop PV, Hobbs R. Aggression in general practice. Br med J. 1989;298:97–8.
77. Myerson S. Under Stress? Practitioner. 1990;234:973–6.
78. Strathdee G, Williams P. A survey of psychiatrists in primary care: the silent growth of a new service. J R Coll Gen Pract. 1984;34:615–8.
79. Katz J. Why doctors don't describe uncertainty in professional judgement. In Dowie J, Elstein A, eds. Professional judgement: a reader in clinical decision making. Cambridge University Press. 1988:544–65.
80. Lief HI, Fox RC. Training for 'detached concern' in medical students. In Lief HL, Lief VF, Lief NR, eds. The Psychological Basis of Medical Practice. New York: Harper and Row. 1963:449–60.
81. Roland MO, Bartholomew J, Courtney MJ, Morris RW, Morrell DC. The five-minute consultation. Br Med J. 1986;292:874–6.
82. Howie JGR, Porter AMD, Forbes JF. Quality and use of time in general practice: widening the discussion. Br Med J. 1989;298:1008–10.
83. Cartwright LK. Continuity and non continuity in the careers of a sample of young women physicians. J Am Med Wom Assoc. 1977;32(9):316–21.
84. Mawardi BH. Satisfaction, dissatisfactions, and causes of stress in medical practice. JAMA. 1979;241:1483–6.
85. Mechanic D. The organization of medical practice orientations among physicians in prepaid and non-prepaid primary care settings. Med Care. 1975;13:189–204.
86. McDonald A, McLean IG. Study of the work of general practitioners. Practitioner. 1971;207:608.
87. Richardson IM, Howie JGR, Durno D, Gill G, Dingwall Fordyce I. A study of general practitioners in North East Scotland. J R Coll Gen Pract. 1973;23:132–42.
88. Howie JGR. Patterns of work. Trends in General Practice. In: Fry J, ed. For the Royal College of General Practitioners by the British Medical Journal, London, 1977:22–35.
89. Howie JGR, Porter AMD. Provision of primary care in the United Kingdom. Oxford Textbook of Public Health. 1985.
90. French J, Caplan R. Organisational stress and individual strain. In Marrow A, ed. The Failure of Success. New York: Amazon. 1972:31–66.
91. Kahn RL, Wolfe DM, Quinn RP, Shock JD, Rosenthal RA. Organisational Stress: Studies in Role Conflict and Ambiguity. UK: John Wiley. 1964:41.
92. Bowling A. Delegation in General Practice: A Study of Doctors and Nurses. London: Tavistock. 1981.
93. Gilmore M, Bruce N, Hunt M. The Work of the Nursing Team in General Practice. Council for Education and Training of Health Visitors, London. 1974.
94. General Practitioner. August 12 1988.
95. Ducker DG. The effects of two sources of role strain on women physicians. Sex Roles. 1980;6:549–59.
96. Wardwell WI, Hyman M, Bahson CB. Stress and coronary disease in three field studies. J Chron Dis. 1964;17:73–84.
97. French JRP, Caplan RD. Psychosocial factors in coronary heart disease. Ind Med. 1970;39:383–97.
98. Cobb S, Rose RM. Hypertension, peptic ulcer and diabetes in air traffic controllers. JAMA. 1973;224:489–92.
99. Jones FA, Doll R, Fletcher CM, Rodgers HW. Risks of gastroscopy. Survey of 49,000 examinations. Lancet. 1951;1:747–51.
100. Russek HI, Sohan BL. Relative significance of hereditary, diet and occupational stress in CHD of young adults. Am J Med Sci. 1960;235:266–75.
101. Rosenman RH, Friedman M, Straus R. CHD in the Western collaborative group study. JAMA. 1966;195:86–92.
102. Margolis BL, Kroes WH, Quinn RP. Job stress: an unlisted occupational hazard. J Occup Med. 1974;1(16):659.
103. Burke RJ, Weir T, Duwors RE. Type A behaviour of administrators and wives' reports of marital satisfaction and well being. J Appl Psychol. 1979;64:57–65.
104. Burke RJ, Weir T, Duwors RE. Work demands on administrators and spouse well-being. Hum Relations. 1980;33:253–78.
105. Sekaran U. Factors affecting the quality of life in dual career families. J Occup Psychol. 1983;56:161–74.
106. Cooke RA, Rousseau DM. Stress and strain from family role and work – role expectations. J Appl Psychol. 1984;67:361–9.
107. Billings AG, Moos RH. Work stress and the stress buffering roles of work and family resources. J

Occup Behav. 1982;3:215–32.
108. Burke RJ, Belcourt ML. Managerial role stress and coping responses. J Bus Admin. 1974;5:55–68.
109. Vaillant GE, Sobowale NC, McArthur C. Some psychologic vulnerabilities of physicians. N Engl J Med. 1972;287:372–5.
110. Scheiber SC. Emotional problems of physicians. I. Nature and extent of problems. Ariz Med. 1977;34:323–5.
111. Fine C. Married to Medicine: An Intimate Portrait of Doctors' Wives. New York: Atheneum. 1981.
112. Werber R. A doctor's wife interviews 100 doctors' wives. Physician Manage. 1980;20(11):63–8.
113. Nelson S. Some dynamics of medical marriages. J R Coll Gen Pract. 1978;28:585–7.
114. Kennie AT. The contribution of doctors' wives to general practice. J R Coll Gen Pract. 1962;12:353–69.
115. Dearlove J, Bate T, Dearlove B et al. Ignoring the obvious: doctors' wives as patients. Br Med J. 1982;285:187–9.
116. Driscoll GL, Fong PS. Obstetric performances in medical marriages, Letter. Lancet. 1982;1:57.
117. Sakinofsky I. Suicide in doctors and their wives. Br Med J. 1980;281:386–7.
118. Barker MG. The doctor's family. Rendle short lecture 1980, April. In the Service of Medicine, Suppl.
119. Bennet G. Patients and Their Doctors. London: Balliere Tindall. 1979.
120. Bird C. The Two Paycheck Marriage: How Women at Work are Changing Life in America. New York: Rawson Wade. 1979.
121. Walton J. Harben Lecture. Illness in doctors and their families. Health Hyg. 1989;10:51–62.
122. Miles JE, Krell R, Lin RY. The doctor's wife: mental illness and marital pattern. International J Psychiatr Med. 1975;6:481–7.
123. Cooper CL, Davidson MJ. High Pressure–Working Lives of Women Managers. London, Fontana. 1982.
124. Social Trends. London: HMSO. 1991.
125. Cooper CL. Executive Families Under Stress. New Jersey: Prentice-Hall. 1982.
126. Roscow I, Rose KD. Divorce among doctors. J Marriage Fam. 1972;34:587–98.
127. Richings JC, Khara GS, McDowell M. Suicide in young doctors. Br J Psychiatry. 1986;149:475–8.
128. Firth-Cozens J. Sources of stress in women junior house officers. Br Med J. 1990;301:89–91.
129. Nadelson CC, Notman MT. What is different for women physicians? In Scheiber SC, Doyle BB, eds. The Impaired Physician. New York: Plenum. 1983.
130. Walsh MR. Doctors Wanted: No Women Need Apply. New Haven: Yale University Press. 1977.
131. Cartwright LK. Career satisfaction and role harmony in a sample of young women physicians. J Voc Behav. 1978;12:184–96.
132. Goode W. A theory of role strain. Am Sociol Rev. 1960;25:473–96.
133. Coser RL, Rokoff G. Women in the occupational world: social disruption and conflicts. Soc Problems. 1971;18:535–54.
134. Heins M, Smock S, Martindale L, Jacobs J, Stein M. Comparison of the productivity of women and men physicians. JAMA. 1977;237(23):2514–7.
135. Nadelson C, Notman M, Lowenstein P. The practice pattern, life styles and stresses of women and men entering medicine: a follow-up study of Harvard Medical School graduates from 1967 to 1977. J Am Med Wom Assoc. 1979;34:400–6.
136. Angell M. Women in medicine: Beyond prejudice. N Engl J Am Med Wom Assoc. 1981;304(19):1161–3.
137. Elliot CM. Women physicians as workers. J Am Med Wom Assoc. 1981;36:105–8.
138. Mandelbaum DR. Work, Marriage and Motherhood: The Career Persistence of Female Physicians. New York: Praeger. 1981.
139. Parkhouse J, Ellin DJ. Reasons for doctors career choice and change of choice. Br Med J. 1988;296:1651–3.
140. Buchan J, Stock J. Early careers of general practitioners. Brighton: Institute of Manpower Studies, University of Sussex. 1990.
141. Gray JP. The doctor's family: Some problems and solutions. J R Coll Gen Pract. 1982;32:75–9.
142. Horder E. Stress in the GP's family. In Royal College of General Practitioners, 1982 Members' Reference Book, London, RCGP.
143. Gabbard GO. The role of compulsiveness in the normal physician. JAMA. 1985;254:2926–9.
144. Robinowitz CB. The physician as a patient. In Scheiber SC, Doyle BB, eds. The Impaired Physician. New York: Plenum. 1983.
145. Bennet G. Sick doctors – ourselves. J Postgrad Med Pract. 1982;24:1621–31.
146. Rosenman RH, Friedman M, Straus R. A predictive study of CHD. JAMA. 1964;189:15–22.
147. Friedman M. Pathogenesis of Coronary Artery Disease. New York: McGraw-Hill. 1969.

148. Friedman M, Rosenman RH. Type A Behaviour and Your Heart. London: Wildwood House. 1974.
149. Jenkins CD. Psychologic and social precursors of coronary disease. N Engl J Med. 1971;284(6):307–17.
150. Jenkins CD, Rosenman RH, Friedman M. Development of an objective psychological test for the determination of the coronary-prone behaviour pattern in employed men. J Chron Dis. 1967;20:371–9.
151. Carruthers M. Hazardous occupations and the heart. In Cooper CL, Payne R, eds. Current Concepts in Occupational Stress. Chichester, New York: John Wiley & Sons. 1980:3–22.
152. Rosenman RH, Jenkins CD, Bland RJ et al. Coronary heart disease in the Western collaborative group study. Final follow-up experience of 8.5 years. JAMA 1975;233:872–7.
153. Bortner RW, Rosenman RH. The measurement of pattern: A behaviour. J Chronic Dis. 1967;20:525–33.
154. Zyzanski SJ, Jenkins CD. Basic dimension within the coronary-prone behaviour pattern. J Chron Dis. 1970;22:781–895.
155. Caplan RD, Cobb S, French JRP. Job demands and workers health. Washington DC: US Department of Health, Education and Welfare Publication No. (NIOSH) 75–160, US Government Printing Office. 1975.
156. Cooper CL. The stress of work: An overview. Aviat Space Environ Med. 1985;July:627–32.
157. McMichael AJ. Personality, behavioural and situational modifiers of work stressors. In Cooper CL, Payne R, eds. Stress at Work. Chichester: John Wiley and Sons. 1978:127–147.
158. House JS. The relationship of intrinsic and extrinsic work motivations to occupational stress and coronary heart disease risk. PhD thesis, The University of Michigan. Reported in Cooper CL, Payne R, eds, Stress at work. 1978. Wiley. 1972.
159. Caplan R. Organisational stress and individual strain: A social–psychosocial study of risk factors in coronary disease among administrators, engineers and scientists. Ann Arbor, Michigan: Research Centre for Group Dynamics. 1971.
160. Rosenman RH. The interview model of assessment of the coronary-prone behaviour pattern. In Dembroski TM, Weiss SM, Sields JL, Haynes SG, Feinlieb M, eds. Coronary-Prone Behaviour. New York: Springer-Verlag. 1978:55–69.
161. Dembroski TM, Caffrey B, Jenkins CD, Rosenman RH, Spielberger CD, Tasto DL. Section summary: assessment of coronary prone behaviour. In: Dembroski TM, Weiss SM, Shields JL, Haynes SG, Feinlieb M, eds. Coronary prone behaviour. Springer-Verlag: New York. 1978.
162. Glass DC, Krakoff LR, Contrada R, Hilton WF, Kehoe K et al. Effect of harassment and competition upon cardiovascular and catecholaminic responses in Type A and Type B individuals. Psychophysiology. 1980;17:453–63.
163. Haynes SG, Feinlieb M. Women, work and coronary heart disease: prospective findings from the Framingham heart study. Am J Public Health. 1980;70:133–41.
164. Waldron I. Sex differences in the coronary-prone behaviour pattern. In Dembroski TM, Weiss SM, Shields JL, Haynes SA, Feinlieb M, eds. Coronary-Prone Behaviour. New York: Springer-Verlag. 1978:199–205.
165. Cooper CL, Davidson MJ. The pressurs on working women: What can be done? Bull Br Psychol Soc. 1981;34:357–60.
166. Davidson MJ, Cooper CL. Type A coronary-prone behaviour in the work environment. J Occup Med. 1980;22(6):375–83.
167. Kasl SV. Mental health and work environment. An examination of the evidence. J Occup Med. 1973;15:506–15.
168. Caplan RD, Jones KW. Effects of workload, role ambiguity and type A personality on anxiety, depression and heart rate. J Appl Psychol. 1975;60:713–9.
169. Cooper CL. Work stress in white and blue collar jobs. Bull Br Psychol Soc. 1980;33:49–51.
170. Davidson MJ, Cooper CL. Shattering the glass ceiling. The woman manager. Paul Chapman Publishing Ltd. 1992.
171. Clarke TA, Maniscalco WM, Taylor-Brown S et al. Job satisfaction and stress among neonatologists. Paediatrics. 1984;74:52–7.
172. Melville A. Job satisfaction in general practice: implications for prescribing. Soc Sci Med. 1980;14A:495–9.
173. McCranie EW, Hornsby JL, Calvert JC. Practice and career satisfaction among residency trained family physicians: a national survey. J Fam Pract. 1982;14:1107–14.
174. Mechanic D. General medical practice: Some comparisons between the work of primary care physicians in the United States and England and Wales. Public Expectations and Health Care. New York: Wiley. 1972.

175. Ryle JA, Russell WT. The natural history of coronary disease: a clinical and epidemiological study. Br Heart J. 1949:11:370–89.
176. Breslow L, Buell P. Mortality from coronary heart disease and physical activity of work in California. J Chronic Dis. 1960;11:615–26.
177. McDonough JR, Hames CG, Stulb SC, Garrison GE. Coronary heart disease among negroes and whites in Evans County, Georgia. J Chron Dis. 1965;18:443–68.
178. Syme SL, Hyman MM, Enterline PE. Some social and cultural factors associated with the occurrence of coronary heart disease. J Chron Dis. 1964;17:277–89.
179. Miles HH, Waldfogel S, Barrabee EL, Cobb S. Psychosomatic study of 46 young men with coronary artery disease. Psychosom Med. 1954;16:955.
180. Russek HI. Role of hereditary, diet and emotional stress in coronary heart disease. JAMA. 1959;171:503–8.
181. Blohmke M, Schaefer H, Abel H, Depner R, Koschorreck B, Stelzer O. Medizinische and Soziale Befunde bei koro-naren Herzkrankheiten. Munch Med Wschr. 1969;III:701–10.
182. Bruhn JC, McCrady KE, Du Plessis A. Evidence of 'emotional drain' preceding death from myocardial infarction. Psychiatr Dig. 1968;29:34–40.
183. Floderus B. Psychosocial factors in relation to coronary heart disease and associated risk factors. Nord Hyg Tidsskr. 1974:6.
184. Medalie JH, Snyder M, Groen JJ, Nenfeld NH, Goldbourt U, Riss E. Angina pectoris among 10,000 men, 5 year incidence and univeriate analysis. Am J Med. 1973;55:583–94.
185. Wilhelmsen L. Stress and coronary heart disease. Aust NZ J Med. 1980;10:135–8.
186. Medalie JH, Kahn HA, Newfield HN, Riss E, Goldbourt U, Perlstein T, Oron D. Myocardial infarction over a five year period. I. Prevalence, incidence and mortality experience. J Chronic Dis. 1973;26:63–84.
187. Shekelle RB, Schneider AS, Liu SC, Raynor WJ, Garron DC, Ostfeld AM, Paul O. Work tension and risk of coronary heart disease (CHD). Am Heart Assoc CVD Epidemiol. News Lett. 1979;26:66.
188. Theorell T, Floderus-Myrhed B. Workload and risk of myocardial infarctions. A prospective psychosocial analysis. Int J Epidemiol. 1977;6:17–21.
189. Kittel F, Kornitzer M, Dramaix M. Coronary heart disease and job stress in two cohorts of bank clerks. Psychother Psychosom. 1980;34:110–23.
190. Sobolski J, Backer G, de Degre S, Kornitzer M, Denolin H. Physical activity, physical fitness and cardiovascular diseases: design of a prospective epidemiologic study. Cardiology. 1981;67:38–51.
191. Dublin LI, Spiegelman M. The longevity and mortality of American physicians, 1938–1942. JAMA. 1947;134:1211–15.
192. Dickinson FG, Martin LW. Physician mortality, 1949–1951 Bureau of Medical Economic Research. J Am Med Assoc. 1956;162:1462–8.
193. Dublin LI, Spiegelman M. Mortality of medical specialists, 1938–1942. JAMA. 1948;137:1519.
194. Office of Population Census and Surveys. Occupational Mortality. The Registrar General's Decennial Supplement for England and Wales (1970–72). London: HMSO. 1978.
195. Williams SV, Munford RS, Colton T, Murphy DA, Poskanzer DC. Mortality among physicians: a cohort study. J Chron Dis. 1971;24:393–401.
196. Everson RB, Fraumeni JF. Mortality among medical students and young physicians. J Med Educ. 1975;50(8):809–11.
197. Goodman LJ. The longevity and mortality of American physicians: 1969–1973. Millbrook Mem Fund Q. 1975;53:353.
198. Doll R, Peto R. Mortality in relation to smoking: 20 years observations on male British doctors. Br Med J. 1976;2:1525–36.
199. Schuckit MA, Gunderson EKE. Job stress and psychiatric illness in the US navy. J Occup Med. 1973;15:884–7.
200. Lancet. Doctors as patients. Editorial. 1983;2:201.
201. Duffy C, Litin EM. Psychiatric morbidity of physicians. J Am Med Assoc. 1964;189:989–92.
202. A'Brook MF, Hailstone JD, McLauchalan IEJ. Psychiatric illness in the medical profession. Br J Psychiatry. 1967;113:1013–23.
203. Vincent MO, Robinson EA, La HL. Physicians as patients: psychiatric hospital experience. Can Med Assoc J. 1969;100:403–12.
204. Pond DA. NZ Med J. 1969;69:131. Cited in Murray RN. The health of doctors: a review. J R Coll Physicians. 1978;12:October.
205. Small IF, Small JG, Assue CM, Moore CF. The fate of mentally ill physicians. Am J Psychiatry. 1969;125:39–47.

206. Franklin RA. 100 doctors on the retreat. Br J Psychiatry. 1977;131:11–14.
207. Jones RE. A study of 100 physician psychiatric in-patients. Am J Psychiatr. 1977;134(10):1119–23.
208. Murray RM. The health of doctors: a review. J R Coll Physicians. 1978;12(5):403–15.
209. Vaillant GE, Sobowale NC, McArthur C. Some psychologic vulnerabilities of physicians. N Engl J Med. 1972;287:372–5.
210. Murray RM. Psychiatric illness in male doctors and controls: an analysis of Scottish in-patient hospital data. Br J Psychiatry. 1977;131:1–10.
211. Bojar S. Psychiatric problems of medical students. In Blaine GB, McArthur CC, eds. Emotional Problems of the Students. New York: Appleton-Century Crofts;1971:350–63.
212. Pitts FN, Winokur G, Stewart MA. Psychiatric syndromes, anxiety symptoms and responses to stress in medical students. Am J Psychiatry. 1961;118:333–40.
213. Salmons PH. Psychiatric illness in medical students. Br J Psychiatry. 1983;143:505–8.
214. Lloyd C, Cartkell NK. Psychiatric symptoms in medical students. Compr Psychiatry. 1984;25:552–65.
215. Firth JA. Levels and sources of stress in medical students. Br Med J. 1986;292:1177–80.
216. Vernon SW, Roberts RE, Lee ES. Ethnic status and participation in longitudinal health studies. Am J Epidemiol. 1984;119:99–113.
217. Bjorksten O, Sutherland S, Miller C, Steward T. Identification of medical student problems and comparison with those of other students. J Med Educ. 1983;58:759–67.
218. Friedman RC, Kornfield DS, Bigger TJ. Psychological problems associated with sleep deprivation in interns. J Med Educ. 1973;48:436–41.
219. Valko RJ, Clayton PJ. Depression in the internship. Dis Nerv Syst. 1975;36:26–9.
220. Waring EM. Emotional illness in psychiatric trainees. Br J Psychiatry. 1974;125:10–11.
221. Werner ER, Adler R, Robinson R, Korsch BM. Attitudes and interpersonal skills during paediatric internship. Paediatrics. 1979;63(3):491–9.
222. Lief VF, Lief HI, Young KM. Academic success, intelligence and personality. J Med Educ. 1965;40:114.
223. Nadelson C, Notman M. Adaption to stress in physicians. In Shapiro E, Lowenstein L, eds. Becoming a Physician. Cambridge: Ballinger Publishing Company. 1979.
224. HMSO. Occupational mortality. The Registrar General's decennial supplement for England and Wales (1970–72). London. 1978.
225. Blackly PH, Disher W, Roduner G. Suicide by physicians. Bull Suicidology. December 1968;1–18.
226. Steppacher RC, Mausner JS. Suicide in male and female physicians. JAMA. 1974;228:323–8.
227. Rose KD, Roscow I. Physicians who kill themselves. Arch Gen Psychiatry. 1973;29:800.
228. Craig AG, Pitts FN Jr. Suicide by physicians. Dis Nerv Syst. 1968;29:763–72.
229. Thomas CB. What becomes of medical students: the dark side. Johns Hopkins Med J. 1976;138:185–95.
230. Sargent DA. Physician suicide. A paper presented at the annual meeting of the American Collge of Psychiatrists, Marco Island. 1986.
231. Scheiber SC. Stress in physicians. In Payne R, Firth-Cozens J, eds. Stress in Health Professionals. Chichester: John Wiley & Sons.1987:23–44.
232. Schwartz AH, Schwartzburg M, Lieb J, Slaby AE. Medical school and the process of disillusionment. Med Educ. 1978;12:182–5.
233. Norwood-East W. British Journal of Addiction. 1949;46:38. Cited in Murray R. J R Coll Physicians. 1978;12(5):415.
234. Bailey RD. Coping with stress in caring. Blackwell Scientific Publications; London. 1985.
235. Irvine D. Reported by Mary Bishop in Family Practitioner. 1982;12:46.
236. HMSO. Report of the Committee of Inquiry into the Regulation of the Medical Profession. Cmnd 6018, London. 1975.
237. Vaillant GE, Brighton JR, McArthur C. Physicians' use of mood-altering drugs: A 20-year follow-up report. N Engl J Med. 1970;282:365–72.
238. Bissell L, Jones RW. The alcoholic physicians: A survey. Am J Psychiatry. 1976;133:1142.
239. A'Brook MF. Psychosing and depression. The Practitioner. 1990:234:992–3.
240. Anslinger HJ. Interview. Mod Med. 1957;25:170.
241. Pescor M. Diseases of the Nervous System. 1942;3:173. Cited in Murray R. J R Coll Physicians. 1978;12:415.
242. Wall JH. Federation Bulletin. 1958;45:144. Cited in Murray R. J R Coll Physicians. 1978;12(5):415.
243. Modlin HC, Montes A. Narcotic addiction in physicians. Am J Psychiatry. 1964;121:358–65.
244. Putnam PL, Ellingwood EH Jr. Narcotic addiction among physicians: a ten year follow-up. Am J Psychiatry. 1966;122:745–8.

245. Green RC, Carroll GJ, Buxton WD. Drug addiction among physicians. The Virginia experience. JAMA. 1976;236(12):1372–5.
246. Hurrell JJ, Kroes WH. Stress Awareness. Cincinnati: National Institute for Occupational Safety and Health. 1975.
247. Hoyland P. Alcoholism affects one person in twenty-five. The Guardian. June. 1980.
248. Cooper CL, Cooper CR, Eaker LH. Living with stress. London: Penguin. 1988.
249. Murray RM. Alcoholism amongst male doctors in Scotland. Lancet. 1976;2:729–33.
250. Lloyd G. I am an alcoholic. Br Med J. 1982;285:785–6.
251. Efron V, Keller M, Gurioli C. Statistics on consumption of alcohol and on alcoholism. Rutgers Centre of Alcohol Studies, New Brunswick, New Jersey, NJ Publications Division. 1974.
252. The Impaired Physician. AMA. Department of Mental Health. Conference on the impaired physician, September 1978.
253. Gomberg ES. Problems with alcohol and other drugs. In Gomberg ES, Franks V, eds. Gender and Disordered Behaviour. New York: Brunner/Mazel. 1979:204–40.
254. McCrae RR, Costa PT, Bosse R. Anxiety, extroversion and smoking. Br J Soc Clin Psychol. 1978;17:269–73.
255. Murray R. The sick doctor. Med Int. 1983;1(34):1582–4.
256. Murray RM. The mentally ill doctor: causes and consequences. Practitioner. 1983;222:65–75.
257. Lee PN. Has the mortality of male doctors improved with the reductions in their cigarette smoking? Br Med J. 1979;2:1538–40.
258. Social Trends. London, HMSO. 1981.
259. Roscow I, Rose KD. Divorce among doctors. J Marriage Fam. 1972;34:587–98.
260. Kasl SV, Cooper CL. Stress and Health: Issues in research methodology. New York: John Wiley & Sons. 1987.
261. Wilkin D, Hallam L, Leavey R, Metcalf D. Anatomy of Urban General Practice. London: Tavistock. 1987.
262. Hale R, Hudson L. The Tavistock Study of young doctors: report of the pilot phase. Br J Hosp Med. 1992;47(6):455–64.
263. Linn LS, Kosecoff J, Clark V et al. Preliminary Evaluation Report: Provider Survey Data, Los Angeles, Report Wood Johnson Teaching Hospital General Medicine Group Practice Program. 1982.
264. Frankenhauser M. Quality of Life Criteria for Behavioural Adjustment. Report from the Department of Psychology, University of Stockholm (No. 475). 1976.
265. Elliot FR. The conflict between work and family in hospital medicine. Health Trends. 1978;10:17–8.
266. De Sole DE, Singler P, Aranson S. Suicide and role strain among physicians. Int J Soc Psychiatry. 1969;15:294–301.
267. Hudson G. Counsellors within general practice: time and need for utilization and accreditation. Counselling Psychol Sec Rev. 1988;3(1):15–20.
268. Gravelle HSE. Deputising Services: Prescribing in General Practice and Dispensing in the Community. London, Kings Fund Centre. 1980.
269. Mitchell J. What Is To Be Done About Illness and Health? Harmondsworth, Penguin. 1984.
270. Pulse. September 16, 1989.
271. Horobin G, McIntosh J. Time, risk and routine in general practice. Sociol Sociology of Health and Illness. 1983;5(3):312–31.
272. Huntington J. Take the stress off your practice. Medeconomics. 1984;5(12).
273. Sibbald B, Addington-Hall J, Brenneman D, Freeling P. Counsellors in English and Welsh general practices: their nature and distribution. Br Med J. 1993;306:29–33.
274. Financial Pulse. February 21, 1989.
275. Financial Pulse. April 25, 1989.
276. Office of Health Economics. Compendium of Health Statistics, 5th edn. London: OHE. 1984.
277. Rawnsley K. Physician, don't heal thyself: let someone else try! Practitioner. 1989;233:891.
278. Myers J, Lindenthal J, Pepper MP. Life events, social integration and psychiatric symptomatology. J Health Soc Behav. 1975;16:121–7.
279. Rahe R, O'Neill TO, Hagan A, Arthur RJ. Brief group therapy following myocardial infarction – eighteen month follow-up of a controlled trial. Int J Psychiatric Med. 1975;6:349–58.
280. Chesney MA, Rosenman RH. Type A behaviour in the work setting. In Cooper CL, Payne R, eds. Current Concerns in Occupational Stress. Chichester: Wiley. 1980:187–212.
281. Gentry WD. Behaviour Modification of the Coronary-Prone (Type A) Behaviour Pattern. In Dembroski TM, Wiess S, Shields JL et al., eds. Coronary-Prone Behaviour. New York: Springer-Verlag. 1978:225–30.

282. Suinn RM. How to break the vicious cycle of stress. Psychology Today. 1976;10:59–60.
283. Benson H. Your innate asset for combatting stress. Harvard Bus Rev. 1974;52:49.
284. Evison R. Effective stress management. Management of inappropriate negative emotions. Occup Psychol. 1988;6:11–21.
285. Medical Monitor. 9th October, 1992.
286. Rice PL. Stress and health, 2nd edn. Brooks/Cole Publishing Company, California. 1992;355.

Appendices

Appendix 1: Questionnaire Forms

SECTION A		Office use only	
Only for the purpose of statistical analysis, would you please answer the following questions about yourself by circling the appropriate response. Your answers will remain anonymous and strictly confidential.			
1. What is your job title	Trainee / Principal	☐	1
2. What is your age	25-34 35-44 45-54 55-64 over 65	☐	
3. What is your sex	Male / Female	☐	
4. Are you	Married / Single		
	Divorced / Separated / Widowed		
	Remarried / Living together	☐	
5. What is your practice type	Solo / Group	☐	
6. Were you qualified in the UK	Yes / No	☐	
If no, how long have you lived in this country	under 1 year		
	1-5 years		
	5-10 years		
	over 10 years	☐	
7. Any post-graduate qualifications	Yes / No	☐	
8. How many years have you spent in General Practice including training	under 10 years		
	10-15 years		
	15-20 years		
	20-25 years		
	over 25 years	☐	
9. Your practice location	Rural / Urban	☐	10

SECTION B

Office use only

Stress or pressure is defined as a problem, something you find difficult to cope with and about which you feel worried or anxious. The greater the pressure the higher the number. Please **circle** the number that best reflects the degree to which the particular statement is a source of stress in your job.

Codes:
1 = No stress at all
2 = A source of slight stress
3 = A source of moderate stress
4 = A source of considerable stress
5 = A source of extreme stress

Item						Office use only	
1. Conducting surgery	1	2	3	4	5	☐	11
2. Home visits	1	2	3	4	5	☐	
3. Night calls	1	2	3	4	5	☐	
4. Dealing with problem patients	1	2	3	4	5	☐	
5. Practice administration	1	2	3	4	5	☐	
6. Hospital referrals and paper work	1	2	3	4	5	☐	
7. Arranging admissions	1	2	3	4	5	☐	
8. Driving in relation to your work	1	2	3	4	5	☐	
9. Emergency calls during surgery hours	1	2	3	4	5	☐	
10. Demands of your job on family life	1	2	3	4	5	☐	
11. Demands of your job on social life	1	2	3	4	5	☐	
12. Dividing time between spouse and patients	1	2	3	4	5	☐	
13. Lack of emotional support at home especially from spouse	1	2	3	4	5	☐	
14. Remaining alert when on call	1	2	3	4	5	☐	
15. Coping with numerous journals and newsletters	1	2	3	4	5	☐	
16. Worrying about patients' complaints (e.g. professional misconduct)	1	2	3	4	5	☐	
17. Daily contact with dying and chronically ill patients	1	2	3	4	5	☐	
18. Taking work home (paper work, referral letters etc.)	1	2	3	4	5	☐	
19. 24 hour responsibility for patients' lives	1	2	3	4	5	☐	
20. Interruption of family life by telephone	1	2	3	4	5	☐	
21. Coping with phone calls during night and early morning	1	2	3	4	5	☐	31

						Office use only	
22. Fear of assault during night visits	1	2	3	4	5	☐	32
23. Taking several samples in a short time (blood, swab, smear etc.)	1	2	3	4	5	☐	
24. Working environment (surgery setup, lack of facilities etc.)	1	2	3	4	5	☐	
25. Conflict with partners in a group practice	1	2	3	4	5	☐	
26. Increased demands by patients and relatives for second opinions from hospital specialists	1	2	3	4	5	☐	
27. Dealing with the terminally ill and their relatives	1	2	3	4	5	☐	
28. No appreciation of your work by patients	1	2	3	4	5	☐	
29. Dealing with friends as patients	1	2	3	4	5	☐	
30. Dealing with relatives as patients	1	2	3	4	5	☐	
31. Examining patients of the opposite sex	1	2	3	4	5	☐	
32. Adverse publicity in the press	1	2	3	4	5	☐	
33. Time pressure	1	2	3	4	5	☐	
34. Unrealistically high expectations by others of your role	1	2	3	4	5	☐	
35. Coping with new technology (e.g. computers)	1	2	3	4	5	☐	
36. Partner on holiday	1	2	3	4	5	☐	
37. Finding a locum	1	2	3	4	5	☐	
38. Visiting in extremely adverse weather conditions (i.e. snow, frost etc.)	1	2	3	4	5	☐	
39. Any other sources of stress?						☐	49
Please state:-____________________ (Continue on last page if necessary)							

SECTION C — Office use only

Could you please **circle** one number for each of the 14 questions below, which best reflects the way you behave in everyday life.

For example, if you are always on time for appointments, on question 1 you would circle a number between 7 and 11. If you are usually more casual about appointments you would circle one of the lower numbers between 1 and 5.

													Office use only
Casual about appointments	1	2	3	4	5	6	7	8	9	10	11	Never late	☐ 50
Not competitive	1	2	3	4	5	6	7	8	9	10	11	Very competitive	☐
Good listener	1	2	3	4	5	6	7	8	9	10	11	Anticipates what others are going to say (nod, attempts to finish for them)	☐
Never feels rushed (even under pressure)	1	2	3	4	5	6	7	8	9	10	11	Always rushed	☐
Can wait patiently	1	2	3	4	5	6	7	8	9	10	11	Impatient while waiting	☐
Takes things one at a time	1	2	3	4	5	6	7	8	9	10	11	Tries to do many things at once, thinks about what to do next	☐
Slow deliberate talker	1	2	3	4	5	6	7	8	9	10	11	Emphatic in speech, fast and forceful	☐
Cares about satisfying him/herself no matter what others may think	1	2	3	4	5	6	7	8	9	10	11	Wants good job recognized by others	☐
Slow doing things	1	2	3	4	5	6	7	8	9	10	11	Fast (eating, walking)	☐
Easy going	1	2	3	4	5	6	7	8	9	10	11	Hard driving (pushing yourself and others	☐
Expresses feelings	1	2	3	4	5	6	7	8	9	10	11	Hides feelings	☐
Many outside interests	1	2	3	4	5	6	7	8	9	10	11	Few interests outside work/home	☐
Unambitious	1	2	3	4	5	6	7	8	9	10	11	Ambitious	☐
Casual	1	2	3	4	5	6	7	8	9	10	11	Eager to get things done	☐ 76

SECTION D	Office use only	
1. Over the past year, which of the following best describes your typical drinking habit? Please circle the appropriate corresponding number.		
Teetotal 0 An occasional drink 1 Several drinks a week 2 Regularly, 1 or 2 drinks a day 3 Regularly, 3-6 drinks a day 4 Regularly, more than 6 drinks a day 5	☐	78
2. Please circle the number which constitutes your average daily consumption of cigarettes.		
None 0 1-10 a day 1 11-20 a day 2 21-30 a day 3 31-40 a day 4 40 plus a day 5	☐	79

SECTION E								Office use only

This set of items deals with various aspects of your job. Would you like to tell us how satisfied you feel with each of these features of your present job. Please use the scale below to indicate your feelings.

Just indicate how satisfied or dissatisfied you are with each of the various aspects of your job by using this scale:-

1 = Extremely dissatisfied
2 = Very dissatisfied
3 = Moderately dissatisfied
4 = Not sure
5 = Moderately satisfied
6 = Very satisfied
7 = Extremely satisfied

Simply **circle** the appropriate number.

Item								Office use only	
1. The physical working conditions	1	2	3	4	5	6	7	☐	1
2. The freedom to choose your own method of working	1	2	3	4	5	6	7	☐	
3. Your fellow worker(s)	1	2	3	4	5	6	7	☐	
4. The recognition you get for your good work	1	2	3	4	5	6	7	☐	
5. The amount of responsibility you are given	1	2	3	4	5	6	7	☐	
6. Your rate of pay	1	2	3	4	5	6	7	☐	
7. The opportunity to use your ability	1	2	3	4	5	6	7	☐	
8. Your hours of work	1	2	3	4	5	6	7	☐	
9. The amount of variety in your job	1	2	3	4	5	6	7	☐	
10. Now, taking everything into consideration, how do you feel about your job as a whole	1	2	3	4	5	6	7	☐	10

SECTION G						Office use only
Please think about the events or situations which have been stressful for you during the last three months. By 'stressful' I mean a situation which was difficult or troubling you, either because it made you feel bad or because it took effort to deal with it. How do you usually cope with these situations? Please **circle** the appropriate response. 1 = Stongly disagree 2 = Moderately disagree 3 = No feelings either way 4 = Moderately agree 5 = Strongly agree						
1. Blamed myself	1	2	3	4	5	☐ 35
2. Kept my feelings to myself	1	2	3	4	5	☐
3. Wished I could have changed what happened	1	2	3	4	5	☐
4. Got mad at the people or things which caused the problem	1	2	3	4	5	☐
5. Let my feelings out in some way	1	2	3	4	5	☐
6. Just concentrated on what I had to do next - the next step	1	2	3	4	5	☐
7. Talked to someone about how I was feeling	1	2	3	4	5	☐
8. Didn't let it get to me; refused to think about it too much	1	2	3	4	5	☐
9. Went on as if nothing had happened	1	2	3	4	5	☐
10. Avoided being with people in general	1	2	3	4	5	☐
11. You went over the problem again and again	1	2	3	4	5	☐
12. Talked to someone who could do something about the problem	1	2	3	4	5	☐ 46

THANK YOU

Appendix 2: The interview sample

Job title	No of GPs	Age range	
Trainee	12	27 – 35	
Principal	30	28 – 60	
Total sample	42		

Sex	No of GPs	Marital status	No of GPs
Male	28	Married	34
Female	14	Single	4
		Divorced	1
		Widowed	1
		Living together	2
Total sample	42	Total sample	42

Qualified from	No of GPs	Practice type	No of GPs
Overseas	15	Solo	7
UK	27	Group	35
Total sample	42	Total sample	42

Practice location	No of GPs
Rural	6
Urban	28
Mixed	8
Total sample	42

Appendix 3: Sex distribution of GPs

Sex	*No.*	*%*	*1970**	*1980**
Male	1469	80.9	90	83
Female	343	18.9	10	17
Total sample	1812			

*Source: Health and Personal Social Services Statistics, 1982

Appendix 4: Age distribution of GPs

Age	*No.*	*%*	*Age**	*%*
25–34	507	27.9	<30	2
35–44	635	34.9	30–	30
45–54	366	20.1	40–	30
55–64	276	15.2	50–	25
Over 65	28	1.5	60–	10
			70–	3
Total sample	1812			

*Source: Health and Personal Social Services Statistics, 1982

Appendix 5: Marital status of GPs

Marital status	*No.*	*%*
Married	1539	84.7
Single	84	4.6
Divorced	40	2.2
Separated	15	0.8
Widowed	16	0.9
Remarried	62	3.4
Living together	49	2.7
Total sample	1805	

Appendix 6: Place of qualification of the GPs

Place of qualification	*No.*	*%*		*1970**	*1980**
UK	1607	88.4	UK & Eire	86	81
Overseas	204	11.2	Elsewhere	14	19
Total sample	1811				

*Source: Health and Personal Social Services Statistics, 1982

Appendix 7: Postgraduate qualification of the GPs

Postgraduate qualification	*No.*	*%*
With PG qualification	1286	70.8
Without PG qualification	522	28.7
Total sample	1808	

Note: The total sample size may vary from variable to variable because of missing cases

Appendix 8: Job demographics of GPs (total sample)

Job	*Sample.*		*1975*		*1982*	
	No.	*%*	*No.*	*%*	*No.*	*%*
Principals	1750	96.5	24644	96.5	27500	93.5
Trainees	63	3.5	882	3.5	1900	6.5
Total sample	1813					

*Source: Personal communication from DHSS, estimated figures

Appendix 9: Practice type of GPs

Practice type	*No.*	*%*
Solo	151	8.3
Group	1657	91.2
Total sample	1808	

Appendix 10: Experience in general practice

Experience in general practice	*No.*	*%*
Under 10 years	787	43.3
10–15 years	369	20.3
15–20 years	211	11.6
20–25 years	150	8.3
Over 25 years	29	16.3
Total sample	1813	

Appendix 11: Practice location of the GPs

Practice location	*No.*	*%*
Rural	339	18.7
Urban	1213	66.8
Mixed	261	14.4
Total sample	1813	

Appendix 12: Job satisfaction (in order of importance)

Dimensions	*Mean*	*SD*
The amount of responsibility you are given	5.68	1.09
The freedom to choose your own method of working	5.40	1.26
The amount of variety in your job	5.38	1.20
Your fellow workers	5.24	1.25
The physical working conditions	5.11	1.41
The opportunity to use your ability	5.04	1.35
Your rate of pay	4.77	1.56
The recognition you get for your good work	4.76	1.18
Your hours of work	4.25	1.57
Overall job satisfaction	5.23	1.15

Range: 1–7, Polarity: Higher score = higher satisfaction

Appendix 13: Distribution of type A scores

	Score range	*No. of GPs*	*%*
Type A1	108 – 154	324	18.08
Type A2	93 – 107	609	33.98
Type B3	64 – 92	795	44.36
Type B4	14 – 63	64	3.57

Appendix 14: Significant differences between GPs and normative groups on type A coronary-prone behaviour

Group	*n*	*Mean*	*SD*	*t*	*p*
Police detective	223	87.6	14.2		
GPs (whole group)	1788	92.94	16.5	5.19	<0.01
Senior male managers	311	69.0	14.5		
GPs (male)	1450	93.09	16.7	27.74	<0.01
Senior female managers	171	73.3	14.9		
GPs (female)	388	92.39	15.79	9.38	<0.01

Appendix 15: Work stressors: highest frequencies: all GPs

Item	*Label*	*Mean*	*SD*
9	Emergency calls during surgery hours	3.48	1.08
3	Night calls	3.45	1.04
21	Coping with phone calls during night/carly morning	3.32	1.12
4	Dealing with problem patients	3.28	0.94
33	Time pressure	3.11	1.07
10	Demands on your job on family life	2.76	1.03
20	Interruption of family life by telephone	2.73	1.09
36	Partner on holiday	2.59	1.04

1 = no stress at all; 5 = a source of extreme stress

Appendix 16: Significant differences between trainee and principal GPs in responses to work stressors

Stressors	*Job*	*n*	*Mean*	*SD*	*t*	*p*
Home visits	T	63	2.41	0.69		
	P	1745	2.19	0.82	2.10	0.036
Taking several samples in a short time	T	63	2.03	0.90		
	P	1740	1.73	0.88	2.71	0.007
Conflict with partners in a group practice	T	63	1.60	0.73		
	P	1680	1.92	1.03	−2.41	0.016
Dealing with terminally ill and their relatives	T	63	2.43	0.80		
	P	1744	2.14	0.90	2.53	0.011
Dealing with friends as patients	T	61	2.61	1.14		
	P	1726	2.22	1.05	2.82	0.005
Dealing with relatives as patients	T	60	2.77	1.27		
	P	1673	2.14	1.19	4.00	0.000
Examining patients of the opposite sex	T	63	1.60	0.85		
	P	1747	1.36	0.61	3.05	0.002
Visiting in extremely adverse weather conditions	T	63	2.62	1.13		
	P	1745	2.26	1.13	2.48	0.013

1 = no stress at all; 5 = a source of extreme stress

Appendix 17: Significant differences between solo and group practice GPs in response to work stressors

Stressors	*Practice type*	*n*	*Mean*	*SD*	*t*	*p*
Conducting surgery	S	149	1.80	0.89		
	G	1653	2.09	2.09	−4.23	0.000
Home visits	S	151	1.99	0.92		
	G	1652	2.22	0.80	−3.40	0.001
Night calls	S	149	3.11	1.11		
	G	1625	3.49	1.02	−4.22	0.000
Dealing with patients	S	151	3.04	1.06		
	G	1649	3.30	0.92	−3.32	0.001
Practice administration	S	151	1.87	0.91		
	G	1643	2.14	0.93	−3.40	0.001
Emergency calls during surgery hours	S	150	2.99	1.27		
	G	1653	3.52	1.05	−5.86	0.000
Demands of your job on family life	S	151	2.60	1.08		
	G	1645	2.76	1.02	−2.06	0.040
Lack of emotional support from spouse	S	148	1.82	1.15		
	G	1618	1.65	0.99	2.01	0.045
Remaining alert when on call	S	151	1.82	1.03		
	G	1636	2.12	1.10	−3.26	0.001
Coping with numerous jounals and newsletters	S	150	1.86	1.00		
	G	1652	2.09	1.05	−2.58	0.010
24 hour responsibility for patients' lives	S	150	2.60	1.27		
	G	1643	2.37	1.13	2.35	0.019
Coping with phone calls during night and early morning	S	150	3.01	1.20		
	G	1643	3.35	1.10	−3.51	0.000
Fear of assault during night visits	S	150	1.97	1.27		
	G	1633	1.75	1.08	2.41	0.016
Conflict with partners in a group practice	S	86	1.41	1.08		
	G	1652	1.93	1.01	−4.68	0.000

1 = no stress at all; 5 = a source of extreme stress

Appendix 18: Dependent variable: mental health – crown-crisp experimental index (CCEI) comparisons of GPs and normative population on CCEI

Group	*n*	*Mean*	*SD*	*t*	*p*
Free floating anxiety					
Female GPs	335	4.84	3.35		
Female population	415	5.40	3.50	−2.23	<0.05
Male GPs	1439	3.70	3.17		
Male population	340	2.80	2.80	5.19	<0.01*
Somatic anxiety					
Female GPs	335	2.65	2.24		
Female population	415	5.70	3.30	−15.02	<0.01
Male GPs	1439	2.36	2.18		
Male population	340	4.30	3.00	−11.24	<0.01
Depression					
Female GPs	335	3.37	2.39		
Female population	415	4.40	2.50	−32.08	<0.01
Male GPs	1439	2.94	2.65		
Male population	340	3.20	2.30	−1.82	NS

The male and female normative data for the CCEI was obtained by Crown–Crisp (1979) on random sample of patients in two large group practices, one in an urban and the other in a rural area (Priest, 1971).
(Polarity: Higher score = lower mental wellbeing)

Appendix 19: Significant differences between UK and overseas qualified GPs in response to work stressors

Stressors	*Place of qualification*	*n*	*Mean*	*SD*	*t*	*p*
Conducting surgery	UK	1601	2.11	0.77		
	Overseas	204	1.71	0.87	7.02	0.000
Dealing with problem patients	UK	1599	3.31	0.90		
	Overseas	204	3.00	1.14	4.45	0.000
Practice administration	UK	1593	2.14	0.92		
	Overseas	204	1.97	1.00	2.43	0.015
Driving in relation to your work	UK	1603	1.45	0.70		
	Overseas	203	1.66	0.89	−3.84	0.000
Emergency calls during surgery hours	UK	1603	3.53	1.04		
	Overseas	203	3.08	1.30	5.54	0.000
Demands of your job on family life	UK	1597	2.79	1.01		
	Overseas	202	2.57	1.12	2.82	0.005
Lack of emotional support from spouse	UK	1570	1.64	0.98		
	Overseas	199	1.82	1.14	−2.34	0.019
Worrying about patients complaints	UK	1601	2.45	1.18		
	Overseas	204	2.69	1.35	−2.75	0.006
Taking work home (paperwork, etc.)	UK	1592	1.93	0.95		
	Overseas	199	2.13	1.08	−2.74	0.006
24-hour responsibility for patient's lives	UK	1593	2.33	1.09		
	Overseas	203	2.85	1.33	−6.16	0.000
Fear of assault during night visits	UK	1583	1.65	0.98		
	Overseas	203	2.69	1.50	−13.33	0.000
Taking several samples in a short time	UK	1600	1.70	0.84		
	Overseas	201	2.04	1.14	−5.32	0.000
Working environment	UK	1602	1.62	0.84		
	Overseas	201	2.80	1.07	−2.71	0.007

1 = no stress at all; 5 = a source of extreme stress

Appendix 20: Significant differences between rural and urban practice GPs in response to work stressors

Stressors	*Practice location*	*n*	*Mean*	*SD*	*t*	*p*
Night calls	Rural	336	3.36	0.96		
	Urban	1187	3.51	1.05	−2.34	0.01
Hospital referral and paperwork	Rural	339	1.99	0.87		
	Urban	1210	1.87	0.88	2.31	0.02
Demands of your job on family life	Rural	338	2.89	0.96		
	Urban	1204	2.72	1.05	2.65	0.008
Demands of your job on social life	Rural	339	2.52	1.05		
	Urban	1207	2.38	1.00	2.17	0.03
Remaining alert when on call	Rural	338	1.98	1.03		
	Urban	1199	2.15	1.11	−2.47	0.01
Worrying about patients complaints	Rural	338	2.37	1.14		
	Urban	1208	2.53	1.22	−2.14	0.03
Interruption of family life by telephone	Rural	339	2.87	1.07		
	Urban	1207	2.70	1.10	2.55	0.01
Coping with phone calls during night and early morning	Rural	339	3.44	1.05		
	Urban	1200	3.30	1.12	2.05	0.04
Fear of assault during night visits	Rural	338	1.46	0.87		
	Urban	1192	1.92	1.16	−6.75	0.000
Taking several samples in a short time	Rural	339	1.67	0.84		
	Urban	1204	1.78	0.90	−2.05	0.04
Working environment	Rural	339	1.55	0.75		
	Urban	1205	1.69	0.91	−2.58	0.01
Increased demands by patients and relatives for second opinions from hospital specialists	Rural	339	2.07	0.96		
	Urban	1212	2.19	0.95	−2.10	0.03

1 = no stress at all; 5 = a source of extreme stress

Appendix 21: Significant differences between male and female GPs in response to work stressors

Stressors	*Sex*	*n*	*Mean*	*SD*	*t*	*p*
Practice administration	M	1460	2.09	0.92		
	F	338	2.26	0.98	−3.01	0.003
Demands of your job on family life	M	1464	2.44	1.01		
	F	342	2.24	0.99	3.36	0.001
Dividing time between spouse & patients	M	1449	2.41	1.08		
	F	303	2.17	1.00	3.35	0.000
Coping with numerous journals & newsletters	M	1463	2.03	1.03		
	F	343	2.21	1.11	−2.85	0.004
Daily contact with dying and	M	1466	2.10	0.90		
chronically ill patients	F	340	2.28	0.86	−3.32	0.001
Interruption of family life by telephone	M	1465	2.76	1.90		
	F	340	2.61	1.08	2.34	0.019
Fear of assault during night visits	M	1462	1.61	0.99		
	F	325	2.48	1.27	−13.63	0.000
Dealing with terminally ill and their relatives	M	1464	2.11	0.89		
	F	342	2.32	0.91	−3.84	0.000
Dealing with friends as patients	M	1456	2.18	1.04		
	F	330	2.46	1.09	−4.35	0.000
Dealing with relatives as patients	M	1420	2.11	1.17		
	F	312	2.40	1.27	−3.86	0.000
Coping with new technology	M	1453	1.93	1.00		
	F	339	2.26	1.03	−5.34	0.000
Partner on holiday	M	1409	2.57	1.04		
	F	329	2.69	1.05	−1.96	0.051
Finding a locum	M	1401	1.97	1.14		
	F	314	2.27	1.22	−4.19	0.000
Visiting in extremely adverse weather conditions	M	1464	2.16	1.11		
	F	343	2.75	1.09	−8.86	0.000

1 - No stress at all; 5 = a source of extreme stress

Appendix 22: Interviews in 1992 (after the introduction of the new contract)

The interviews were carried out in the north-west region. The areas were selected by us but the GPs within each area were chosen randomly from the local FHSA lists. After initial contact by telephone 49 out of the sample of 60 GPs were interviewed. This gave a response rate of 81.67%. The main reason for not being able to interview all GPs contacted initially was due to their lack of time.

Interviews were conducted by us between June 1992 and September 1992, with 49 GPs; 36 male and 13 female.Interviews took place in the surgeries and each interview lasted from 30 to 50 minutes. The interview format was unstructured at the beginning but as a result of the response of the interviewees became more structured. Nevertheless, discussion of any other points raised by the doctors was encouraged.

Useful addresses and telephone numbers

The Professional Counselling Group: 0494-722455

National Counselling Service for Sick Doctors
3rd Floor
26 Park Crescent
London
W1N 6AE
Tel: 071-580 7642

British Association for Counselling
37A Sheep Street
Rugby
Warwickshire
CV21 3BX
Tel: 0788-578328

MIND (National Association for Mental Health)
22 Harley Street
London
W1N 2ED
Tel: 071-637-0741